BEYOND CARROTS

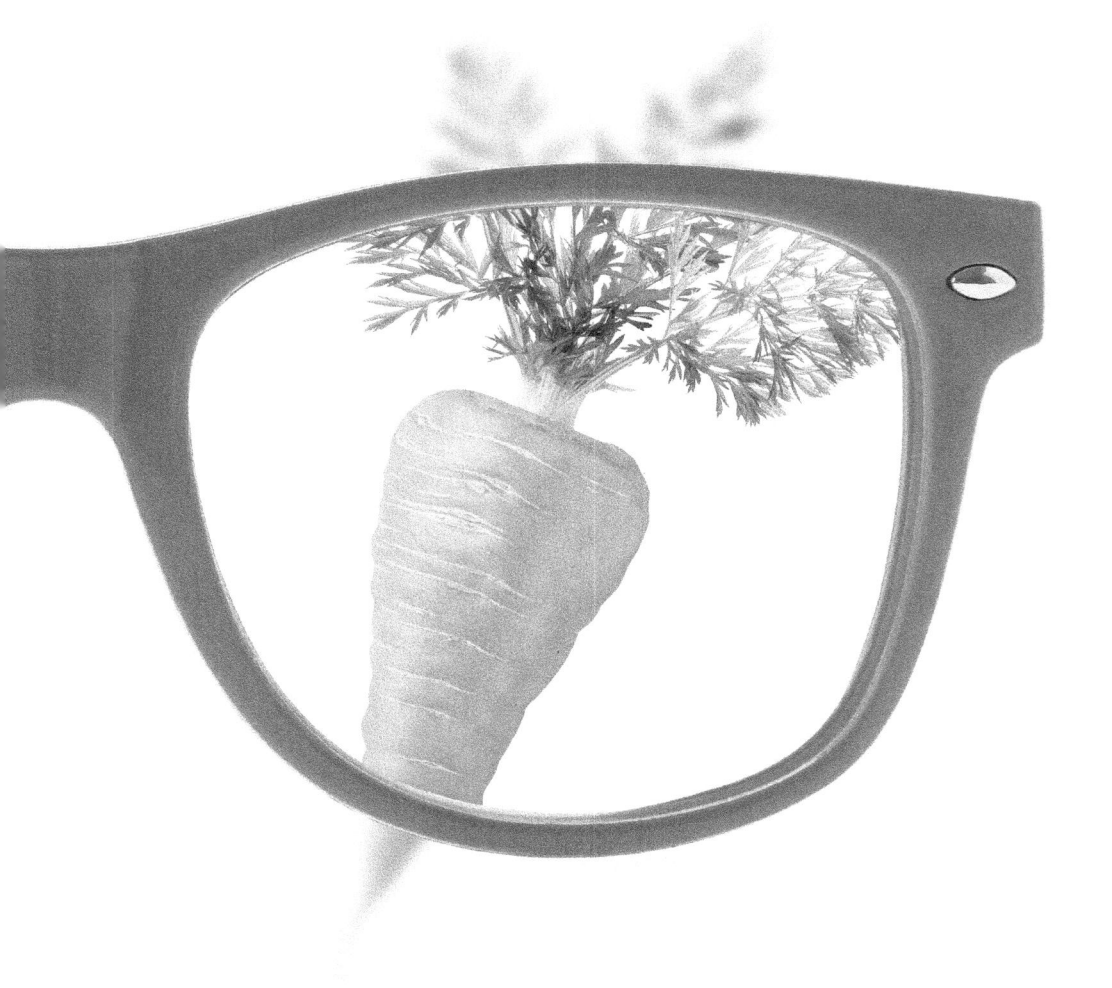

Eye disease can happen to you too

DR. BRITNEY CARUSO

BEYOND CARROTS
Copyright © 2022 Dr. Britney Caruso. All rights reserved.

No part of this book may be used or reproduced in any manner whatsoever without written permission, except in the case of brief quotations embodied in critical articles and reviews. For more information, e-mail all inquiries to info@mindstirmedia.com.

Published by Mindstir Media, LLC
45 Lafayette Rd | Suite 181| North Hampton, NH 03862 | USA
1.800.767.0531 | www.mindstirmedia.com

Printed in the United States of America
ISBN-13: 979-8-9861392-0-3

BEYOND CARROTS
Eye disease can happen to you too

Dr. Britney Caruso

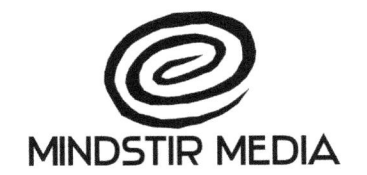

MINDSTIR MEDIA

Table of Contents

Chapter 1: Eye Disease… It Can Happen to Anyone
- Introduction — 7
- The Scariest Day Ever — 8
- Our Journey Together — 11

Chapter 2: Crash Course in Ophthalmology
- Structure of the Eye, Minus Scientific Mumbo Jumbo — 14
- Why Glasses, Contacts, and LASIK Don't Always Work — 17
- How 99% of Eye Diseases Start — 19

Chapter 3: Eye Diseases and How They Can Be Impacted by Food and Lifestyle
- Cataracts: The World's Leading Cause of Blindness — 21
- Macular Degeneration: How 5 Millimeters of Your Eye Can Impact Your Life — 30
- Dry Eye: The Oxymoron — 35
- Glaucoma: You Can't Smoke Weed in Your Sleep — 42
- Diabetes, Obesity, and Hypertension: The Three Stooges — 48
- Uveitis: A Big Word for Inflammation — 55

Chapter 4: What to Eat and What to Avoid
- Gut Health: Your First Line of Defense — 60
- Gluten: But I Don't Have Celiac Disease So I Can Skip this Chapter…Wrong! — 66
- But I Thought Tomatoes, Bell Peppers, and Zucchini Are Vegetables? — 72
- Other Potential Culprits — 74
- What is White, Grainy, and More Addictive than Cocaine? — 76
- An Apple a Day Keeps the Doctor Away — 78
- What do British Fighter Pilots and Carrots Have in Common? — 82
- Popeye Was a Smart Man — 83
- The Anti-Cancer Food — 84

- The Pee-You Power — 87
- Battle of Land and Sea — 89
- America Really Does Run on Coffee! — 91
- Jewish Penicillin — 94
- What Color is Your Urine — 96
- How To Drink Like an Italian — 98

Chapter 5: Lifestyle and Its Impact on Eye Health
- A 60 Hour Work Week Can Actually Cause Vision Loss. Tell That to Your Boss — 103
- If You Can Walk Your Dog, You Can Meditate — 105
- God, Allah, Buddha, I Don't Care — 106
- Did You Know Shopping Is Exercise? Now That Does Not Sound So Bad, Does It? — 108
- Vitamin D vs. UV Light — 110
- Get Those Zzz's — 113
- It is Long, White, and Skinny and Kills Just About Every Bone in Your Body — 117

Chapter 6: Beyond Carrots Plan
- The Two Beyond Carrots Plans — 119
- Beyond Carrots Plan Step 1: Mentally Prepare — 121
- Beyond Carrots Plan Step 2: Baseline Testing — 124
- Beyond Carrots Plan Step 3: Spring Cleaning — 134
- Beyond Carrots Plan Step 4: Planning for Success — 137
- Beyond Carrots Plan Step 5: Get Out Those Tupperware Containers — 147
- Beyond Carrots Plan Step 6: KISS Vitamins — 150
- Beyond Carrots Plan Step 7: Get Off Your Butt — 153
- Beyond Carrots Plan Step 8: Take 10 — 156
- Beyond Carrots Plan Step 9: Assess Your Progress — 157
- Beyond Carrots Plan Step 10: Reward Yourself — 159
- Baby Steps Beyond Carrots Plan — 161

Conclusion: I Am SOOOOO Grateful — 167

Bibliography

Chapter 1:
Eye Disease ... It Can Happen to Anyone

Introduction

I bet you picked up this book thinking that, maybe, just maybe, it may help to reverse your eye disease. But what about all of those people out there who do not necessarily have eye disease? Great news! This book is for ALL of you, too! There is one thing I want you to take away from this book. Your eyes are connected to your body. Anything that you put in your body, do to your body, or feel with your body affects your eyes. This is incredibly powerful in so many ways. For starters, we can actually change the fate of our eye health by making simple modifications in our behaviors. Secondly, we can look into the eyes and tell what is going on in the body. How amazing is that! If you do not believe me, just wait till you see what I have in store for you. This stuff will blow your socks off.

To take things one step further, there is a reason why the eye doctor is considered a primary care physician. The eye doctor is often the first person to find diseases that are running rampant throughout the body. This is because the tiny blood vessels in the back of the eye are fragile and super susceptible to damage from diseases like diabetes and high blood pressure. This is why it has become mandatory for all diabetic patients to get an eye health evaluation. The health care community is doing its best to keep a good handle on diabetic eye problems because twelve out of a hundred new cases of blindness are related to diabetes. This number is staggering!

Diabetes is just one example of how diseases affect the eye. Rheumatoid arthritis is another classic disease that has eye complications galore. Researchers estimate that 25 percent of those people with rheumatoid arthritis will have eye problems ranging anywhere from dry eye to retinal detachment. Diabetes and rheumatoid arthritis are not isolated incidences of unique cases where the body and the eyes are connected. Regardless of your condition, the eyes are along for the ride.

My goal is to raise awareness of the importance of a thorough eye evaluation by telling you a brief story about the scariest day of my life. Then, I will go on to tell you about how medical diseases, nutrition, and lifestyle can impact your eye health. We will conclude with a plan on how to reverse your eye disease using diet and nutrition. The *Beyond Carrots* Plan will go beyond the eyes and help change every aspect of your health, leaving you feeling healthier and seeing better with documented metrics to measure your success.

The Scariest Day Ever

I graduated high school at the top of my class and went off to Boston College where I graduated with *cum laude* honors. By the time I crossed the stage with my Doctor of Optometry from the Illinois College of Optometry, I felt like I had conquered the world! Literally, everything that I had worked so hard to achieve in my life had come to fruition, and there was no problem that I could not handle. Life could not have been better! Then, I had the scariest day of my life.

At the age of thirty-five, I had been practicing optometry for about ten years and was an officer of the Palm Beach County Optometric Association. I was diligent about maintaining my Pilates and yoga practices, eating healthy, and swimming nearly six miles a week. I saw my medical doctor annually with a clean bill of health. I was feeling pretty good about life because I felt established and secure.

As an officer of my local optometry association, I was a key figure at our association's largest annual convention. My duty was to thank all of the vendors who contributed so much time and energy to the conference. I made my way around the room to a booth that had an extraordinary camera that took a clear picture of the entire back part of the eye. The vendor asked me if I would like to take a picture of my eye so that I could see how well the camera worked. I was like, "Sure, why not?"

When they took the picture of my eyes, I could not believe what I saw.

I said, "This cannot be the picture that you just took." They insisted that it most definitely was a picture of my eyes. The vendor could not understand why I was so upset because although they could take the picture, they didn't know how to interpret the image. However, I instantly knew that I would probably be blind in the near future. There were nine blood spots in one eye and seven in the other. These sixteen blood spots had the power to change my life.

The Monday morning after the conference, I immediately sent the photos of my eye to an ophthalmologist and asked him to please let me know if he agreed with me about what I saw in the images. He said that he could barely see the blood spots, and it was "probably nothing to worry about."

That answer did not quite settle right in my stomach, so I went to an ophthalmologist who focused specifically on the retina. This specialist ordered a regular retina photo to be taken. He took one look at my retina photos and told me once again that he saw no blood spots. I asked him to continue looking at the hemorrhages as they would not be visible in that picture; he needed a widefield camera.

After completing the full retina evaluation, he agreed that there were some hemorrhages and requested that his technicians perform a fluorescein angiography. During this test, the doctor shoots dye in the arm with an IV then looks to see what happens within the ten minutes that it takes for dye to travel through the arm and all the way up to your eye. When this test was done, we found that most of the back part of my eye was leaking fluid, and a substantial amount of my eye was not receiving any blood supply.

This was very concerning because when you do not have a blood supply to any area, your body reacts by creating new blood vessels. This sounds good, but it isn't! The blood vessels are very weak and, if they break in the eye, you can go blind. The doctor told me that it was a very good thing that I came to the clinic that day because if we didn't stop the bleeding, I would most likely be blind within months.

I had been studying and looking at eyes for almost fourteen years but, for the first time, I understood the value of eyesight. The thought of losing vision was devastating. My mom was in the exam room with me when my suspicions became reality. The yellow-stained tears from fluorescein dye dripped down my cheeks. I could not have been more depressed, and what does a woman do when she is depressed? Go shopping!

Mom and I left the doctor's office and made a straight shot to Worth Avenue in Palm Beach! I could barely see to read when I picked out a watch. My mom said that she thought it was a really dumb purchase because she knew in just a few months, I probably wouldn't even be able to read the time.

I am proud to say I now wear that watch every day as a reminder of the most pivotal day of my life.

I proceeded to see every type of medical doctor from rheumatologists to endocrinologists and was eventually diagnosed with idiopathic peripheral retina vasculitis of autoimmune origin. It is an extremely rare condition. Put simply, my body was attacking my eyes. In order to stop the attack, I was put on oral prednisone, which would calm the immune system. In addition, my doctor lasered about the back part of my eye three separate times to kill off the area of my eye that was not receiving any blood supply so that new blood vessels would not form.

I was on prednisone for about six months and could not remain on it any longer because it can cause a number of medical problems, including but not limited to osteoporosis, early cataract formation, and excessive weight gain. My medicine was then switched to methotrexate, an anti-cancer medication that has been used to treat a number of conditions such as rheumatoid arthritis and a skin disease called psoriasis. At this point, I was at the end of my rope with the oral medications, and I knew about the detrimental effects that they could have on the body. This medicine would also put a damper on enjoying a glass of wine now and then as it has toxic effects on my liver.

About five days after starting this last medication, I was awake all night with thoughts of how this medication was affecting my body, and I was concerned about how I was going to cope with my future blindness. I then began praying that God would point me in a direction that would help me heal my eyes. I spent the rest of the night and the next day trying to figure out what I could do to help fix my eyes. When I finally had my plan in place, I was glowing and smiling ear from to ear because I was positive that I had the answer to my eye problem. The biggest problem that I faced at this time was convincing my retina specialist to take me off the oral medications so that I could test out my non-conventional treatment approach. My doctor said that he would agree to give me just thirty days to try my approach, but if it did not work, he would have to put me back on medication.

I admit that the protocol that I had created to fix my eye disease was definitely not easy, but the threat of facing blindness was even worse. The two things I look forward to the most every day are my coffee in the morning and red wine in the evening. In my plan, I had to eliminate all alcohol and coffee for the entire thirty days. In addition, I was to eat only foods that grew in and on the ground, eliminate all nightshades (tomatoes, eggplants, peppers), and stay away from beans.

I also made some lifestyle changes. For instance, I began to meditate daily, which was not as easy as it sounds because getting me to stay in one place for more than a minute and a half is next to impossible. Yoga has always been a big part of my life, but I practiced it a bit more over the course of the next thirty days. I also turned to God and asked for his help in my healing process, so I can't take all the credit.

I went back to my ophthalmologist thirty days after starting my non-conventional approach with a feeling of accomplishment. I was proud of myself for setting out to do something and following through even though it was difficult. I was hopeful that I would hear good news that day.

Guess what?

My plan was a success! There was no leakage of fluid from my blood vessels, and my eyes healed 100 percent! Everyone in the clinic was amazed. Several doctors came in to see the results of my tests because they had heard about my unique case and could not believe that the hemorrhaging would cease with nutrition and lifestyle.

I knew that I had done something amazing and must share my knowledge with as many people as possible. So, I decided at that very moment that I was going to become a specialist in nutrition and eye health, and I got a Fellowship in Metabolic and Nutritional Medicine and was board certified as a member of the American Board of Anti-Aging Health Practitioners with the American Academy of Anti-Aging Medicine (A4M). In fact, I am one of three optometrists in the nation with these certifications.

I look at my experience and my knowledge in this subject matter as a blessing that I must share. I was at church during the Super Bowl weekend this year, and the pastor talked about sharing our gifts with everyone. God gave me the gift of sight, knowledge to share, and the ability to communicate. I thank God for his presence in my life, and I hope to help improve the lives of as many people as possible.

Our Journey Together

In order to be successful at anything you do, you must have a clear understanding of where you are and where you are going. Our journey together will not be three to five hours, or however long it takes for you to read this book. Our journey together is going to be one that lasts a lifetime.

Take a moment to think about your answers to the following questions:
1. Have you been diagnosed with a potentially blinding eye condition? If so, what is the condition?
2. Is someone in your family suffering from blindness?
3. What are your goals in reading this book?
4. Do you have healthy eyes but looking to improve vision?
5. What do you currently eat for breakfast, lunch, and dinner on a typical day? (Be as detailed as possible.)
6. Would you consider yourself physically active? How many minutes of physical activity do you get on a daily basis?
7. How many minutes a day do you meditate and/or pray?
8. How would you rate your quality of sleep?
9. If you could change one aspect of your life, what would it be?

Throughout this book, we will answer every one of those questions. Before we do so, we go through a crash course in ophthalmology. Included in this course is a detailed talk about the meaning of "inflammation," with some critical analogies to understand before you move on to learning how to control or reverse eye disease.

Next, we talk about some of the most common eye diseases that could affect anyone with a short description of the disease process followed by how to modify diet and lifestyle to control or reduce the risk of further development. Although this is not a comprehensive list of all eye diseases, pretty much every reader will face a minimum of one of these diseases at some point in your life.

This is what you have all been waiting to hear! Here we discuss what to eat and what to avoid. We discuss hot topics in nutrition and wellness, and I help you create a plan to reduce eye disease that will work for you. It is my opinion that eating plans are not one size fits all. I am here to give you the knowledge and resources to decide what you want to do to optimize your health.

Lifestyle is something that very few people realize relates directly to eye health. Here we talk about the simple lifestyle changes that can have a powerful impact on your eye health. I bet you did not realize that you can actually go blind from stress. Now you realize why this is one of the most important sections of the book. Do not skip it!

In the final part of the book, we put it all together with the how-to guide. Remember, this is YOUR plan with YOUR goals. I will give you the knowledge and resources and what you do with it is up to you. In the *Beyond Carrots* Plan, we will go through a step-by-step plan to execute the goals you have created while reading this book. I guarantee that if you do every step in this plan, you will see a measurable improvement. Every four weeks, you will review your achievements, recenter your mindset, and push towards higher goals. For that reason, this is not a book that you will let gather dust on your bookshelf.

I will tell you that I am incredibly disciplined, hard-working, and knowledgeable about nutrition and anti-aging medicine, and I find myself occasionally slipping back into old habits. I am no angel! Living a healthy lifestyle is not easy. I am in the trenches with all of you. Just because I wrote the book does not mean that I do not understand the struggles we go through to be healthy. For that reason, there is a *Beyond Carrots* community where we can lean on each other for support on our website, www.beyondcarrots.com, and on our FaceBook page. We need to support one another in our journey to the healthiest lives possible.

Chapter 2:
Crash Course in Ophthalmology

Structure of the Eye, Minus Scientific Mumbo-Jumbo

Before I start telling you about various foods and their impact on your eye health, we have to take a step back and make sure you understand some of the basics about eye structure and how the eye works. First, I will break down each part of the eye and tell you how it functions using the most basic terminology.

Human Eye Anatomy

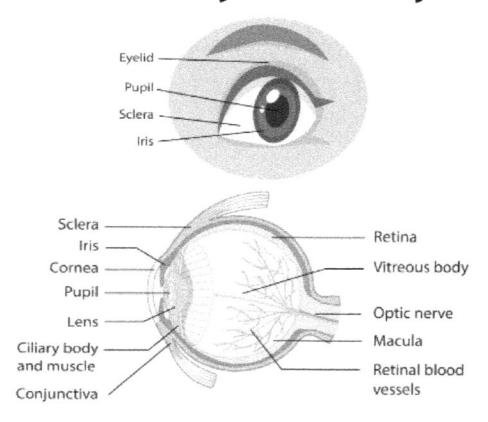

Eyelids: The eyelids function as windshield wipers that help disperse tears and wash away debris from the eyeball. For example, just like your car squirts water and your windshield wipers wash away bird poop from your windshield, your eyelids wash away debris from the front part of your eye. The eyelids also help to keep the front part of the eye moist. If someone has a condition that prevents the eyelids from closing completely, like a face-lift gone bad, the front part of the eye will dry out, and they will suffer reduced vision, pain, and discomfort from the dryness.

Meibomian glands: If you look very closely at the tip of your lid with a magnifying glass, you will probably see tiny holes in a line across the lid margin. These holes are attached to the meibomian glands, which produce oil that helps keep the tears from drying up super quickly. If these oils do not flow out of the holes freely, your tears evaporate as quickly as they are produced, and you will experience dryness. In addition, if these holes become blocked, you may see a big red ball form on the front of your lid called a stye or chalazion, which can be very uncomfortable.

Lacrimal gland: The lacrimal gland is like a water tank that produces and stores tears. It is located just underneath the outer part of your eyebrow. There is a steady flow of tears from the lacrimal gland across the eye lid all day long. However, if you get something in the eye or if the eye is irritated, the brain tells the eye it needs to open the water tank and flush the eye with tears. This is a great defense mechanism because it will quickly get debris off the eye and onto the cheek. However, there are times that your eye may feel like there is something in it, but there really isn't anything there, so excess tears are produced.

Cornea: Keeping on with the windshield analogy that we started with the eyelids, your cornea is the windshield that you look through when you are driving your car. If you have a crack in your windshield right smack dab in your line of sight, you will have difficulty seeing to drive. Likewise, if you have a problem on the cornea like a scratch, you will have difficulty seeing properly. This structure must be crystal clear for your vision to be as clear, and the smallest distortion in the cornea can significantly impact your vision. Your eye is like a tiny camera, and the cornea is one of the "lenses" in the camera that helps focus the picture on the back part of the eye. The cornea is one of the fastest healing structures in your body. Often, the entire cornea can regenerate in as few as 24–48 hours!

Iris: The iris is the colored part of the eye that contracts and expands when exposed to light. The black hole at the center of the iris is called the pupil. I bet you did not realize that the act of expanding and contracting is actually a defense mechanism that is linked to our "fight or flight" response. When you are exposed to something potentially dangerous, your pupils expand to allow the most amount of light in so that you can see more to fight off the potential danger. Likewise, when you are relaxed while watching a movie, the pupil size may not be quite as large. In a similar manner, when your eyes are exposed to light, your pupil size shrinks, and when placed in a darker room, the pupil size expands. When the doctor puts drops in your eyes to evaluate the health of the back part of the eye, the medication in the drops helps to make the pupil large so that the doctor can see through the opening of your eye and evaluate the back part of the eye.

Lens: The lens is like a big magnifying glass that focuses light from the cornea on the back part of the eye. This structure is composed of tons of perfectly aligned proteins so that the vision is as clear as possible. If these proteins become damaged or shift out of alignment, the vision can be affected. When lots of these proteins start aging, your lens gets very cloudy. This is what is commonly referred to as a cataract.

Ciliary muscles: Ciliary muscles are a group of muscles that surround the lens of the eye. When you are trying to read or see something up close, these muscles pull out their big guns and help you focus. When you are trying to see something far away, these muscles relax. The act of moving from seeing something far away to seeing something up close is called accommodation.

Aqueous: The fluid in the front part of the eye that surrounds the lens and the back surface of the cornea is called aqueous. The root of the word "aqueous" is water. You can think of this as a puddle of water in the front part of the eye. But this is an important puddle because it helps deliver key nutrients to the important areas of your eye. So, keeping the right amount of aqueous in this area is critical. Too much water in this area is a big problem as it can contribute to a potentially blinding eye disease called glaucoma.

Vitreous humor: The vitreous humor, otherwise known as the vitreous, is a big ball of jelly in the back of the eye that helps the eye keep its shape. It is made of collagen, just like your ears and nose, but the collagen in the vitreous humor is arranged in a way that keeps it clear so that light can travel through it and hit the back of the eye. All the collagen particles must be arranged as perfectly as soldiers in the army. If one of these collagen soldiers steps out of sequence, you could have an obstruction in your vision, commonly known as a floater.

Retina: The retina is the back part of the eye where light focuses. If we were to consider the eye to be like a camera, the retina would be the film where the image is made. Ironically, everything appears on the retina flipped and inverted, but our brain learns how to process the images during our first six months of life. The retina is composed of several layers of nerves and tiny blood vessels. Because the eye's blood vessels are so small and fragile, they are one of the first areas of your body to be affected by most diseases. When the nerves of the eye are stimulated, you perceive light. Here is a fun experiment, close your eye and gently press on your eyeball. You may see flashes of light even though there is clearly no light hitting the back part of the eye. The physical stimulation is being perceived as light flashes by the brain.

Optic nerve: The optic nerve is a direct extension of the brain, and it carries all the information from the nerve cells in the back part of the eye off to the brain. Information must travel the entire length of the optic nerve, and the eyes must communicate with each other properly for the image to be processed. A roadblock anywhere on that pathway can affect your ability to see. There is one spot in the back of the eye where the optic nerve leaves the eye and goes to the brain. This one spot has no light receptors and therefore has no vision. For that reason, the area where the optic nerve leaves the eye and goes to the brain is called the "blind spot."

Why Glasses, Contacts, and LASIK Don't Always Work

We need to cover the eye's four major eye conditions that result in the need for glasses. The four conditions that I am talking about are myopia (nearsightedness), hyperopia (farsightedness), astigmatism, and presbyopia. As I said earlier, you are not going to be able to throw your glasses and contacts in the garbage and say you have eagle eye vision without the need for correction on account of the plan you create using this book. These conditions are a result of the shape of your eyeball and the strength of the eye muscles.

In the case of nearsightedness, otherwise known as myopia, the eyeball is too long. Whatever you are trying to see focuses in front of the retina. The big magnifying glass that we call the lens of the eye is working super hard in these eyes. Myopia got the name nearsighted because, in general, people with myopia can see up close without glasses.

Hyperopia (farsightedness) is a result of the eye being too short. In this case, the lens of the eye is not quite strong enough, so what we are trying to see lands behind the retina, and things are blurry. To fix this, we need to give the lens of the eye a little boost with plus-powered glasses that help move the image from behind the back part of the eye onto the retina. Hyperopia acquired the name farsightedness because many people with Hyperopia can see far away without glasses. However, this rule does not always hold true, so if you have a plus-powered prescription, you may find yourself wearing glasses more often than strictly for reading tasks.

Astigmatism is a bit different than myopia and hyperopia in that it can affect both up close and far away vision. Astigmatism often results from the curvature of the cornea. Almost everybody has some degree of astigmatism. Even if your eye doctor did not mention anything about astigmatism during the eye exam, you probably have just little astigmatism. Please do not be concerned about the diagnosis of astigmatism. I promise this is not a fatal diagnosis. If you have a significant amount of astigmatism, it is important that you bring the glasses you have been wearing for years to the eye exam. The doctor is not "cheating" when they look at your old prescription. This information is very important because small changes in your astigmatism can make you feel extremely uncomfortable.

Presbyopia is the last type of problem that we fix with glasses which affects pretty much everyone over the age of forty. Okay . . . let me guess . . . you know someone who is over the age of forty who does not need glasses to read? How did I know you were thinking that? Chances are, that person who is over the age of forty and does not need glasses to read has one of three things going on. It is possible that this person needs glasses to see far away and is not wearing the glasses. There is also a chance that this person just has super-duper strong eyes, and the need for reading glasses has not set in yet. Don't worry; it will set in sooner or later. Lastly, your friend may just not read too much or may be so hardheaded that they are denying the fact that they are getting older and may be procrastinating the dark cloud of the big B-word: bifocals . . . ick!

Now I am going to completely throw you off and tell you that your diagnosis of myopia, hyperopia, astigmatism, and presbyopia, along with the exact amounts of the prescription, may differ when you see different doctors. Yes, it sounds crazy, but it is totally true. Finding the prescription for your glasses is like baking a cake. Three bakers can be given the same ingredients but will probably make three entirely different cakes.

The glasses prescription that is attained during the eye exam is merely the opinion of the eye doctor about what lenses are needed to give you the best possible vision. Different doctors have different opinions and different ways of testing your vision, so it is quite likely that three different doctors on the same day would come up with different glasses prescriptions to give you the best possible vision. At the end of the day, as long as you can see and you are comfortable without strain or headaches, then the eye doctor did a great job.

Although we cannot eliminate the need for glasses and contacts through diet and lifestyle, there are a number of conditions that affect the prescription in your glasses and contacts. As you improve the health of your body and eyes, your prescription may change. A classic example of a shift in your glasses prescription is in the case of diabetes. If you have been diagnosed with diabetes and your blood sugar levels are out of control, you may find that as you stabilize your blood sugar levels, your prescription in glasses and contacts may change.

Now that you understand what glasses, contacts, and LASIK are meant to fix, let's talk about why they don't always work. Sometimes the reason why you cannot see well is because of an eye problem like bleeding in the back part of your eye or a scratch on the front part of your eye. In either of these cases, it is possible that you could put the strongest glasses in the world on, and you still would not have clear vision. The vision is only as good as the eyes are healthy. In order to have the best possible vision with glasses on, your eyes must be as healthy as possible.

How 99 Percent of Eye Diseases Start

At the root of 99 percent of diseases in the body and eyes is inflammation. I know that sounds like an incredibly bold statement, but if you control inflammation, practically all other conditions in your body and eyes will start to resolve. Some of the most common conditions that are directly linked to inflammation are any condition that ends in "-itis."

So, rheumatoid arthritis, dermatitis, optic neuritis, and gastritis are just a few examples of the conditions that end in "-itis" and are inflammatory. Other conditions range from diabetes and hypertension to attention-deficit disorder (ADD)/attention-deficit/hyperactivity disorder (ADHD) and migraines. Over and over again, you will hear me say that conditions are linked to some inflammatory process, so it is critically important for you to understand what this devil of a term "inflammation" really means.

Now that I just got done telling you how horrible inflammation is, I will tell you that some degree of inflammation is necessary for your survival. When you fall and scrape your knee, you see that the area becomes red, irritated, swollen, and hot to the touch. You are experiencing discomfort because the body is sending its fighter cells to the area exposed to the outside world to ensure no infection and keep the bad bacteria from entering the body. THIS IS A GOOD THING! Without inflammation and the hard work of our fighter cells, we would not be able to defend ourselves against the harmful agents that our bodies contact.

Inflammation becomes a bad thing when the fighter cells in our body get confused about what they should be attacking. As a result, these cells end up attacking various parts of the body by mistake. Although you cannot see the swollen, red, inflamed internal organs affected by this mistake attack, the body's systems are affected, which is why we experience various diseases.

Your next question should be, "How can we make sure that we limit mistake attacks?" Excellent question! To understand the answer to this question, let's think about Woodstock. If we were to break our bodies down to the very tiniest particles, we would find these tiny molecules that are surrounded by electrons. Think of electrons as the clothes that surround and protect the molecule. These electrons are critical to keeping everything in check.

Now think about the oxygen that is essential for our survival as a little deviant stinker-pot who likes to party just a little too much. When the party animal, oxygen, is exposed to certain foods, chemicals, or ultraviolet radiation, it acts a little crazy and starts pulling off the electrons from our molecules, so they end up running around without their "clothes" on like the free radicals from Woodstock. This process is known as oxidative stress.

This is where the policemen, antioxidants, come in to help try to control everything. We are trying to combat the oxidative stress that creates free radicals by the deviant oxygen; therefore, the name "anti-oxidant" or "against oxygen" kind of makes sense. The antioxidants are there to tell the free radicals to put their clothes back on and stop causing so much commotion. However, if, by chance, the policemen are not around and the free radicals are allowed to continue partying, we put stress on our bodies, and our systems are impacted in a process called oxidative damage. Because the eyes use more energy than most of the rest of the body, it is the most susceptible organ to oxidative damage.

Some of the most effective antioxidants are vitamins A, C, E, and D. You may consider the acronym ACED, as in, "I ACED that test," to remember these critical vitamins. We will talk extensively about how to control inflammation in the upcoming chapters. You need to understand this process, and you will find out how it is linked to practically every problem in your body.

Chapter 3:
Eye Diseases and How They Can Be Impacted by Food and Lifestyle

Cataracts: The World's Leading Cause of Blindness

Every single person reading this book will either get cataracts themselves or know someone who will get cataracts. Cataracts are, by far, one of the most common eye conditions that enters my exam room. Cataracts affect eighty million people worldwide. A study in 2010 showed that cataracts caused one-third of all blindness worldwide and has been called the world's leading cause of blindness. You may have heard of macular degeneration and glaucoma. Well, there are more people with cataracts than macular degeneration and glaucoma combined. Now that's a pretty compelling reason to read about how to reduce your risk of getting cataracts!

What the Heck are Cataracts Anyway?

Do you recall our discussion of the lens of the eye in the crash course on ophthalmology? The lens is the structure of the eye that is behind the cornea and surrounded by water. The lens of the eye is like the lens of a telescope. It focuses the light of whatever you are looking at on the back part of your eye. To do this, the lens of your eye needs to be clear and flexible. Unfortunately, the lens gets cloudy and rigid as you get older, so you have more difficulty seeing. This cloudy lens is called a cataract.

The lens is made up of tons of proteins that are perfectly aligned, making this structure clear as glass. Any damage to these proteins causes them to clump. I am sure you can imagine that if the proteins bunch up, they are not clear anymore. The hazy lens that results from this clustering of proteins is called a cataract.

It is important for you to understand how the lens of the eye gets its nutrition. For any of the cells in our body to survive, they need nutrients and antioxidants. The majority of our body gets its nutrients from the blood. The lens of the eye is unique in that it has absolutely no blood vessels. You are probably thinking, how can anything survive without blood? Thank God for the water around the lens because this is where it gets all of its nutrition. One reason cataracts develop is that the body of water that surrounds the lens has changes in its nutrients content.

How Do I Know If I Have Cataracts?

I am going to tell you something that you may not believe. Pretty much everyone over the age of sixty has some sort of lens change. The cataracts may be mild, and you may not even feel like your vision is affected. That being said, you are probably not going to go blind overnight so take a deep breath. Part of the reason why cataracts are the world's leading cause of blindness is that many underdeveloped nations do not have the ability to perform procedures necessary to correct cataracts. We are fortunate in America to have many resources to evaluate and manage cataracts in most cases.

If you have cataracts developing, you may notice some of the following:
- Blurred vision
- Double vision
- Glare or "halos" around lights
- Colors do not look as bright
- Difficulty seeing at night
- Need for more light to read

Although they occur more frequently as you get older, cataracts can come at any age. In fact, I am forty-three years old right now, and I have cataracts from the use of steroids to treat my eye condition. This is a perfect example of how the long-term use of certain medications can cause early cataract formation. In addition, you have an increased risk of cataract development if you have certain diseases like diabetes or heart disease. Although we could go on and on with symptoms and risk factors, the best way to know if you have cataracts forming is by going to your eye doctor and getting a complete eye exam.

What Can We Do to Reduce Our Risk of Getting Cataracts?

Eat those oranges! Remember my acronym ACED for some of the most important antioxidants, vitamins A, C, E, and D? Vitamin C becomes important as we talk about cataract formation. This vitamin is water-soluble, which means it dissolves in water. The water that surrounds the lens of the eye carries the vitamin C to the lens. It is interesting to note that there is an age-related decrease in the amount of vitamin C in the lens that is related to cataract formation.

To briefly rehash the importance of vitamin C and antioxidants, let's go back to our Woodstock analogy. Vitamin C is like a policeman that keeps everything in check. If the policemen go away, all order will disappear. When this happens, the tissues are damaged, and cataracts result. We can slow this process if we have enough vitamin C around the water surrounding the lens. The question is, how much vitamin C is enough to keep the free radicals in check?

A study took data from over 110,000 people prior to 2007 and analyzed it to see the role of vitamin C in cataract development. They found that taking 135 mg of vitamin C per day would reduce the risk of cataract development. In the Nutrition Vision Project, they found that women under sixty years old who took 363 mg/day of vitamin C had a 57 percent reduction of cataract formation compared to those who took 140 mg/day. Furthermore, they found that women who took vitamin C for at least ten years had a reduced risk of cataract development.

Based on these studies, I would recommend consuming around 300 mg of vitamin C per day. This sounds like a lot, but it is totally doable by eating the right foods. You could also supplement with vitamins, but, in my opinion, you are always better off getting your nutrients from food.

The chart below is straight from the United Stated Department of Agriculture, Agricultural Research Service, Food Central website.

Food	Milligrams (mg) per serving	Percent (%) DV*
Red pepper, sweet; raw, ½ cup	95	106
Orange juice, ¾ cup	93	103

Food	Milligrams (mg) per serving	Percent (%) DV*
Orange, 1 medium	70	78
Grapefruit juice, ¾ cup	70	78
Kiwifruit, 1 medium	64	71
Green pepper, sweet; raw, ½ cup	60	67
Broccoli; cooked, ½ cup	51	57
Strawberries, fresh; sliced, ½ cup	49	54
Brussel sprouts; cooked, ½ cup	48	53
Grapefruit, ½ medium	39	43
Broccoli, raw, ½ cup	39	43
Tomato juice, ¾ cup	33	37
Cantaloupe, ½ cup	29	32
Cabbage; cooked, ½ cup	28	31
Cauliflower; raw, ½ cup	26	29
Potato; baked, 1 medium	17	19
Tomato; raw, 1 medium	17	19
Spinach; cooked, ½ cup	9	10
Green peas, frozen; cooked, ½ cup	8	9

As you look through the chart, you will find that it is really not that difficult to eat 300 mg of vitamin C from food sources alone. There are more fruits than vegetables at the top of this list, but I would recommend a mix of fruits and vegetables to have the most balanced diet. Broccoli, Brussel sprouts, and cauliflower have made their way onto this list. These foods have some superpowers that we will talk about later.

Vitamin A/Retinol: The Thanksgiving Treat That Can Help Reduce Progression of Cataracts

Two researchers took records of almost 10,000 people to determine the link between vitamin A, otherwise known as retinol, and cataract development. They knew that vitamin A was another one of those key antioxidants that helped keep our body in check, and they thought that maybe they would find a link between this nutrient and cataract formation. What do you know! Those people who had the highest levels of vitamin A in their blood had a reduced risk of developing some of the most common types of cataracts. A second researcher determined that those who took vitamin A supplementation had reduced the risk of developing some types of cataracts.

The big takeaway from these studies is that there is a good chance that eating foods rich in vitamin A can help to reduce your risk of cataract development. You notice that I talk about foods instead of just taking vitamin A in the form of a supplement. I am a firm believer in trying to get as much of these vitamins from food as possible. Here is a list of the foods highest in vitamin A from the United Stated Department of Agriculture, Agricultural Research Service, Food Central website.

Selected Food Sources of Vitamin A

Food	Micrograms (mcg) RAE per serving	Percent DV*
Beef liver; pan-fried, 3 ounces	6,582	731
Sweet potato; baked in skin, 1 whole	1,403	156
Spinach; frozen, boiled, ½ cup	573	64
Pumpkin pie; commercially prepared, 1 piece	488	54
Carrots, raw, ½ cup	459	51
Ice cream, French vanilla; soft serve, 1 cup	278	31
Cheese, ricotta; part skim, 1 cup	263	29
Herring, Atlantic; pickled, 3 ounces	219	24
Milk, fat-free or skim, with added vitamin A and vitamin D; 1 cup	149	17
Cantaloupe; raw, ½ cup	135	15
Peppers, sweet, red; raw, ½ cup	117	13
Mangos, raw; 1 whole	112	12

Breakfast cereals, fortified with 10 percent DV of vitamin A; 1 serving	90	10
Egg; hard-boiled, 1 large	75	8
Black-eyed peas (cowpeas); boiled, 1 cup	66	7
Food	Micrograms (mcg) RAE per serving	Percent DV*
Apricots, dried, sulfured; 10 halves	63	7
Broccoli; boiled, ½ cup	60	7
Salmon, sockeye; cooked, 3 ounces	59	7
Tomato juice; canned, ¾ cup	42	5
Yogurt, plain, low fat; 1 cup	32	4
Tuna, light; canned in oil, drained solids; 3 ounces	20	2
Baked beans; canned, plain, or vegetarian; 1 cup	13	1
Summer squash, all varieties; boiled, ½ cup	10	1
Chicken, breast meat and skin; roasted, ½ breast	5	1
Pistachio nuts, dry roasted; 1 ounce	4	0

Being that beef liver is not at the top of my grocery list, the one food that jumps out to me on this list is sweet potatoes. It is incredible that sweet potatoes have three times as much vitamin A in them compared to spinach or any other food on this list, excluding beef liver . . . ick! So, throw some sweet potatoes on your plate a couple of times a week to get some of the vitamin A that you need to help reduce cataract development. One of the fun things about sweet potatoes is that there are so many ways to eat them. They can range from being a snack as sweet potato fries to serving them as a dessert as sweet potato pie. So, have fun with this cataract-fighting rock star of a food.

Protein: Some of the Most Compelling Research

We can take the data from some massive studies—the Blue Mountain Study of 4,888 people and the European Prospective Investigation into Cancer and Nutrition (EPIC) study of 27,670 people—to evaluate the effects of protein consumption on cataract development. This is where we get some of the most compelling information about how to reduce the progression of cataract growth. These studies found that when people consume ninety-nine grams of protein per day, they had a 50 percent reduction in risk of cataract formation compared to those with lower protein consumption. However, too much of a good thing is no good because, in the EPIC study, it was found that too much protein consumption could actually increase the risk of cataract growth. The moral of the story is that if we keep the amount of protein that we eat per day between 100–125 grams, we could dramatically reduce the risk of cataract development.

Let's take a moment to talk about the sources of protein. The EPIC study breaks down the sources of protein to meat, fish, and vegetables. Interestingly, they found that eating less meat was loosely correlated to less cataract formation. They also found that people sixty-five and older who ate fish and vegetables had a 23 percent reduction in cataract formation. Furthermore, this study revealed that vegetarians of all ages had a reduced risk of cataract development.

It is not up to me to tell you whether to eat only meat, fish, vegetables, or anything in between, but I will tell you that I believe a combination of these foods seems like the way to go. As it relates to cataract formation, loading up on vegetables and eating more fish than meat is a good bet.

Carbohydrates: The Big Word for Sugar

Most of us have heard over and over that we need to be careful with how many carbohydrates we consume because carbohydrates make you fat. The first thing that most people think of when they think of carbohydrates is pasta. It is true that pasta is high in carbohydrates, but so are many healthy foods such as quinoa, bananas, and sweet potatoes. Carbohydrates are just a big word for sugar because carbohydrates are broken down to sugar when you eat them, which raises the amount of sugar in your blood.

It has been found that those people with the lowest level of blood sugar immediately upon waking up in the morning had the lowest cataract development. I am not telling you to eliminate carbohydrates because if we did, we would die. Instead, I would suggest eating nutrient-rich foods and low in carbohydrates to moderate your blood sugar level. The worst time of the day to load up on this energy-producing food is right before bed, as you will not burn as much of that energy in your sleep as you will during the day.

Smoking: This Is Not Rocket Science. Smoking Is Just Bad.

I am going to keep the smoking section short and sweet. I think it has been drilled into our heads how bad smoking is for our health. As it relates to cataracts, smoking drains the body of the antioxidant policemen, which increases cataract formation. Just quit now.

Sunlight Exposure: Pull out Those Shades

Sunlight has all sorts of ultraviolet radiation that is potentially toxic to your skin and your eyes. The form of ultraviolet radiation that is most toxic to the eye's lens is UV-B rays in sunlight. These rays are damaging to the proteins of the lens and can cause cataracts. Let's look at the Salisbury Eye Evaluation Project that had 2,520 people, and the Waterman Study, which evaluated 838. We can take the data from these studies to look at sunlight and its effects on cataract growth.

From this data, it was found over the course of years, the toxic effect of the UV-B light builds up and can cause cataracts to form. Cataracts do not form overnight when your eyes hit sunlight. However, if you do not wear sunglasses with ultraviolet protection from an early age, the damaging effects of the sun will accumulate, and cataracts will be the end result.

Treatment: What Can I Do About These Cataracts?

The good news is cataracts are super easy to treat! First and foremost, get an eye exam. Even if you are not sure if you have cataracts, you should be getting your eyes examined annually by a local optometrist. You may find that you have cataracts, and a simple change in your glasses prescription is all you need to get the best vision. At this visit, your eye doctor may recommend a coating on your glasses' lens that helps reduce the amount of glare that you experience as a result of the cataract called an anti-reflective coating.

If you get your glasses with an anti-reflective coating and you are still slightly unhappy with your vision, you could always consider simply adding additional lighting to whatever you are trying to read or just making the font bigger. You may try these simple changes and find that your lifestyle is being affected by your vision, or you are just not happy with the way you are seeing. In that case, it is time to see your ophthalmologist and consider cataract surgery. This very simple procedure takes no more than seven minutes per eye and has been done millions of times. During cataract surgery, the old, cloudy lens in your eye is removed, and a new, clear lens is put in its place. You will only have to do this procedure once in your lifetime as the new lens will last a hundred years or more. There is, typically, no downtime and you will be up and running the next day. The best part about it is that you can talk to your ophthalmologist about possibly choosing to eliminate the need for glasses after cataract surgery. If I were given a menu with a list of eye problems, cataracts would be my eye problem of choice as it is easy to fix, and I would probably end up being glasses-free after the cataract surgery.

Macular Degeneration:
How Five Millimeters Can Impact Your Life

Can you believe that we use only five millimeters of our eye to see pretty much everything? This important area of the eye is called the macula. Damage to the macula can cause significant vision loss. A condition known as macular degeneration is the leading cause of blindness in the United States and England. The macular degeneration diagnosis can be very scary to an individual because it may feel as if the outlook is dismal. Recent research has unveiled some excellent nutritional tools to help reduce the risk of progression of macular degeneration.

How Do I Know If I Have Macular Degeneration?

Ultimately, the best way to know if you have macular degeneration is to get an eye exam. You could have no change in eyesight but still have the very start of this potentially blinding disease. If you are symptomatic, you may experience blurred vision, difficulty recognizing faces, difficulty tracking words when reading, and vision loss affecting central vision. If you experience any of these symptoms, see your eye care professional immediately for a complete eye exam.

What are the Different Types of Macular Degeneration?

There are two main types of macular degeneration, namely, dry and wet. Dry macular degeneration is by far the most common. Only about 10 percent of macular degeneration cases are wet. Let's back up and talk about what wet and dry actually mean. Wet macular degeneration is termed wet because the macula is wet with fluid that accumulates underneath the back part of the eye.

On the other hand, in dry macular degeneration, there are deposits on the macula. These lumps on the macula distort the vision. In general, vision loss from dry macular degeneration is not as severe as the wet form of this disease.

Macular degeneration is not an all-or-nothing diagnosis. A patient with a mild form may not even be symptomatic. I cannot overemphasize the importance of early diagnosis because natural intervention is most effective before the damage is severe.

What Puts Me at a Higher Risk of Developing Macular Degeneration?

Age: Thus, the name, age-related macular degeneration. Your risk for the disease increases exponentially with elevated age.

Family History: If you have someone in your family with macular degeneration, you are at increased risk of developing this blinding eye disease.

Smoking: Smoking increases your risk of so many things; macular degeneration is no exception.

Race: Caucasians are more likely to get macular degeneration than African Americans or Hispanics.

Obesity/Cardiovascular Disease: People who are obese and have cardiovascular disease have lots of inflammation in their bodies, putting them at increased risk for developing macular degeneration.

Women: Women are at slightly higher risk of developing macular degeneration than men.

So, is the Age-Old Myth That Carrots are Good for Your Eyes Actually True?

When I tell my patients that I am writing a book on nutrition and eye health, the first question that I always get is, "Are carrots really good for your eyes?" Well, here is the big answer that you have all been waiting anxiously awaiting.

Drum roll, please . . .

YES! There is some truth to the fact that carrots are good for your eyes! Whether they reverse blindness is a stretch, but we will go into great detail on why in just a bit. I must tell you, however, that the concept of eating carrots to improve your eyesight was popularized by the British during World War II. You see, the British had pioneered night vision technology to combat the Germans in the night sky. To mask their discovery, they attributed their excellent night vision to the fighter pilot's diet that was supposedly full of carrots. This had a two-fold benefit, it encouraged people to eat a healthy food in a time of famine, and it helped to hide their discovery from their opponents during the war. My grandpa, a POW/MIA in Germany during World War II, would be happy that I knew that fun fact.

Getting back to my initial point, carrots are definitely good for your eyes! If you ever had a picture taken of the back part of your eye, you would notice that the macula, which is the area of the eye used for straight-ahead vision, is reddish-orange. As you work your way to the very center of the best central vision part of the back part of the eye, the colors actually get deeper. If you have a diet rich in colorful foods like carrots, spinach, kale, and sweet potatoes, the pigment in this central part of the eye that aids in our vision increases. Some medical facilities have devices that can measure this amount of pigment in the macula, giving us a measurement called macular pigment ocular density (MPOD).

Who the heck cares about how much pigment you have in the back part of your eye? We all should! Numerous studies reveal that an increase in the macular pigment ocular density has been associated with a reduced risk of developing age-related macular degeneration.

Furthermore, researchers have found that people who have a higher MPOD reading can actually see better! As you improve your eye health, you improve your brain health and cognition. Your eyes are a direct connection to your brain. In a study of over 4,500 Irish people over the age of fifty as part of the Irish Longitudinal Study on Aging, researchers found that the people with the lowest MPOD scores also had worse memory and poorer cognition. Bottom line, the amount of pigment in this five-millimeter zone of the back part of the eye has an incredible impact on your brain and eye function.

Let me try to explain why this pigment is so important to your eye health. When you were a kid, did you ever use a shine the light of the sun through a magnifying glass onto a paper to start a fire, or was I the only naughty kid on the block? (Disclaimer, I was actually a good kid. I did not misbehave until I moved to Fort Liquordale.) Regardless, the light rays through a magnifying glass can start a fire on a piece of paper!

Now think about your eye. The lens of your eye is like a super-strong magnifying glass. Can you imagine how much damage it is doing to the macula every day? The pigment in the macula acts as a sort of superpower sunglasses to protect the macula from the damaging effects of the light rays that hit it and reverse the damage that does occur using its powerful antioxidant strength. More specifically, the pigment in the eye is most effective at absorbing the light before it damages our precious eyes.

Based on all we have covered so far, you may have already figured out that the key to protecting eye health is increasing the MPOD. The fastest and easiest way to increase MPOD is by eating foods rich in a nutrient called carotenoids. Carotenoids are rich in foods that are yellow, orange, and red and function to help absorb light and fight against offenders as they are antioxidants. I bet you noticed that the root word in carotenoids sounds much like carrots. It should not be a surprise that carrots are high in beta-carotene, which is a carotenoid.

There are two main types of carotenoids: carotenes and xanthophylls. We already touched on carotenes like the beta-carotene found in carrots. For the purposes of discussing the eye, the xanthophylls are, arguably, the more important of the two types of carotenoids because they are what we find in the macula. The two xanthophylls that are found in the highest concentration in the macula are lutein and zeaxanthin.

It is also important to give zeaxanthin's cousin, meso-zeaxanthin, some acknowledgment. Meso-zeaxanthin has gotten less credit because it was traditionally deemed the non-dietary xanthophyll as it is not present in plants, but newer research shows that you can actually find meso-zeaxanthin in the skin of fish. You can find the highest level of lutein and zeaxanthin in green leafy vegetables such as kale and spinach and some cruciferous vegetables such as broccoli. Some spices such as basil and parsley are also very high in these phytonutrients.

No discussion about eye vitamins would be complete without talking about the two key studies that unlocked so much of what we know about eye vitamin supplementation. Despite the fact that there are still many unanswered questions, the results of these studies are pretty compelling. The first study is the Age-Related Eye Disease Study, better known as AREDS. In this massive study, researchers looked at how a combination of vitamins and minerals—including vitamin C, E, beta-carotene, and zinc—would impact the risk of development of eye disease such as macular degeneration and cataracts over about six years. They found that these vitamins could reduce the developing advanced age-related macular degeneration by about 25 percent over five years.

In a second study called AREDS 2, researched wondered if including lutein and zeaxanthin along with omega-3 fatty acids would further reduce the progression of advanced macular degeneration. In AREDS 2, they removed beta-carotene from the mix because they found that beta-carotene was linked to the development of lung cancer in smokers. This study found that they could remove beta-carotene and include lutein and zeaxanthin in the formulation and still protect the macula from macular degeneration. Many of the formulations of eye vitamins that are currently on the market follow the AREDS 2 study in their nutrient composition.

When we dive into the "Keep It Simple Stupid Vitamin" chapter, you will learn that I do not encourage taking a ton of vitamins. I believe the majority of our nutrition should come from food. I will help you create a meal plan that will include foods to protect your eyes as part of the *Beyond Carrots* program. That being said, to ensure that you consistently provide your body with the nutrients to protect your eyes, brain, and body, it is best to supplement with an eye vitamin that follows the AREDS 2 results that we just discussed.

Dry Eye: The Oxymoron

Do you know how many times I hear my patients ask, "But my eyes are tearing so much, how are they possibly dry?" Herein lies the oxymoron of dry eye syndrome. Although it may be called dry eye syndrome, one of the hallmark symptoms is excess tearing.

Dry eyes seem like such an innocuous problem. One would think that dryness is not blinding, so it is not that big of a deal. However, dry eye is a very serious problem. First of all, the number of people affected by dry eye disease is staggering. A large study out of China revealed that approximately one-third of people between the ages of five and eighty-nine have some symptoms of dry eye disease. What makes matters worse is that there is a strong correlation between dry eye and depression.

Another study of 3,500 people showed that dry eye leads to a higher depression score than any of the other major eye problems. So, there are many people being affected by this problem, and the people who are affected are often psychologically impacted.

What are the Symptoms Associated with Dry Eye Disease?

1. Tearing: We have already talked about this symptom. Remember that tearing can happen in one or both eyes and still be linked to dryness.
2. Foreign body sensation: Your eyes feel gritty or like there is a piece of sand on the eyeball.
3. Burning/pain: Because the nerves are so close to the surface of the clear part of the eye, when the eye is dry, there is a burning, painful sensation.
4. Redness: Where there is irritation in the body, there is usually redness.
5. Light sensitivity: Dry eye oftentimes results in damage to the cornea. When the eye's windshield is damaged, the light does not enter the eye properly, and there is light sensitivity.
6. Blurred vision: Another result of the cornea being damaged is some

level of blurred vision. It is astonishing how much of an effect dryness can have on the vision. I have seen patients' eyesight improve five visual acuity lines just because they use the dry eye treatment regimen that we will discuss later.

What are Tears Made of? (Boring, I Know, but We Have to Talk about It)

There are three layers to the tear film. The layer that is closest to the cornea is the inner mucin layer. This layer is mucusy and sticky like a big gooey booger. Water loves this layer, so it sticks to it. This facilitates the even spread of water across the entire front surface of the eye.

The middle layer of the tears is called the aqueous layer. This watery layer of the tears is made in the lacrimal gland located under the outer part of your eyebrow. The cornea receives much of its nutrition from this watery layer of tears. The aqueous layer also acts as our front line of defense against anything trying to invade the front part of our eye. If a tiny bug or piece of dust lands on the front of the eye, it is the watery layer of the tears that destroys it or washes it away into the sink hole of our eye called the punctum which is located in the corner near the nose. You can see this hole at the corner of the upper and lower lid in the mirror if you gently pull down on the lid.

The top layer of the tears is called the outer lipid layer. This oily later is produced by the meibomian glands located along the edge of your lid. This layer helps to keep the tears around longer by preventing evaporation. It serves as an additional protective barrier between the eye and the outside world.

What Causes Dry Eye Syndrome?

The single biggest cause of dry eye syndrome is inflammation. I told you that the big I-word was going to be an underlying theme throughout our discussions. If you have been diagnosed with any medical condition associated with inflammation or an autoimmune disease, you are at elevated risk for developing dry eye syndrome. Rheumatoid arthritis, multiple sclerosis, and even diabetes have links to increased eye dryness. Various medications can also lead to increased dryness. Antihistamines, decongestants, and antidepressants are the most common culprits. Story of our lives, you fix one problem and cause another.

Another cause of dry eye syndrome is a problem with the lids. For instance, if the lids do not close properly at night, then the front part of the eye is exposed and will dry up by the morning. In addition, nerve damage, as in polio or Bell's palsy, may cause an inability of one of the eyes to close, which can cause your eyes to dry up.

Let me preface this next statement with the fact that I am not telling you not to get LASIK. LASIK is a great option for the right candidate, but anyone who undergoes LASIK should understand the nerves on the front of the eye are severed in this procedure. If the top layer of cells in the eye cannot feel anything, you blink less, and your body does not know when to produce tears because it never feels dry. As a result, the eye dries up more quickly.

I could go on and on with all the causes of dry eyes. The list is beyond the scope of this book, but I think it is important to touch on some of the environmental causes of dry eye disease. Dry air in a dry climate or on an airplane naturally dries up the eyeball. Likewise, a fan or wind will also quickly dry up the front of the eye. Too much work on the computer can also cause your eyes to dry up quickly. Good news! There are some simple ways to mitigate these problems that we will discuss.

My Dry Eye Treatment Protocol

Over the years, I have created the Caruso Eye Care Dry Eye Treatment Protocol that seems to work. My treatment plan uses minimal medication, and I refer out if the patient needs a procedure to correct the dryness. Although this is definitely not a one size fits all plan, the first thing that I do when I see that a patient has dry eyes is to try to figure out the root cause of the dryness. I practically interrogate my patients to get to the nitty-gritty of what's going on that may be causing the discomfort. Some of the things I address are the following:

Medication/smoking: The easiest first step in treating dry eye is to stop smoking and discontinue any unnecessary medication. There are a number of medications that can be drying to the eyes, such as antihistamines and antidepressants. You should never discontinue medications without discussing your plans with your physician first. If you can survive without a medication, and your doctor is okay with you stopping them, give it a try and see if your eyes feel better. You do not have to get approval from your physician to stop smoking! I am positive you will get their thumbs up on that one!

Consume more water: Sometimes simple is best. Before you start taking a ton of eye drops or modifying your work environment, make sure that you are drinking enough water on a daily basis. You would be surprised by how much water consumption can impact your eyes. Studies show that if you do not drink enough water, you will have drier eyes. So, make sure that you drink approximately sixty-four ounces of water daily before going crazy with drops and other lifestyle changes.

Environment: My next recommendation would be to make simple modifications to your environment. For instance, sleeping with a fan or air conditioning vent hitting you right in the face can dry out the eyes. Taking a minute to reposition the air vents near the bed and in your office workspace can be a simple fix to the dry eye problem.

Another simple environmental change that can reduce dry eyes is adjusting the position of your computer. Believe it or not, your eyes dry up when you spend a lot of time doing work on the computer. The reason for this is two-fold. First of all, you tend to blink less when you concentrate on something. In addition, if the computer is at or above eye level, you have to open your eyes wider to see the computer screen. Moving the computer to approximately 20–30 degrees below eye level allows the lids to close slightly more, resulting in less dryness.

Sleep: The next step is to make sure that you are getting adequate sleep. There is a significant correlation between lack of sleep and several medical conditions ranging from diabetes to heart disease. Dry eyes are one of the many results of poor quality and inadequate sleep.

You may think, well, I don't have much control over my sleep. WRONG! There are many easy things to do to help make sure you get a more restful night of rest. Stress reduction techniques, including deep breathing and meditation, are excellent tools to improve sleep quality. Alcohol consumption also affects sleep patterns. Believe it or not, there are a couple of warm, fuzzy drinks such as bone broth and chamomile tea that help you sleep. So put down the late-night coffee and try one of these delights! We will discuss sleep in greater detail later. The takeaway here is to make sure you are getting the right amount of good quality sleep as a part of the treatment for dry eye syndrome.

Fish oil/omega-3 fatty acids: Another recommendation I give my patients in an effort to reduce dry eye is to make sure they are consuming adequate omega-3 fatty acids. You are going to get so sick of hearing about fish oil and omega-3 fatty acids! Based on my clinical experience and research, I have found that taking approximately 2,000-3,000 mg of omega-3 fatty acids daily for three to six months reduces dry eye syndrome. A number of studies support the use of omega-3 fatty acids in the treatment of dry eye syndrome. One study took the results of seventeen clinical trials with almost 3,500 people and compared the use of omega-3 fatty acids to placebo and found that the use of omega-3 fatty acids resulted in significantly less dryness.

The main reason why fish oil is so effective at reducing dry eyes is that it reduces inflammation in two structures: the lacrimal gland and the meibomian glands. Therefore, more of the watery and oily layers of the tears are produced. The moral of the story is, it may take about three to six months, but consistently taking 2,000-3,000 mg (that is two to three grams) of omega-3 fatty acids daily will result in less inflammation in your eyes and, therefore, less dryness.

Warm compresses: The next super easy step to reducing dry eyes is taking a washcloth and soaking it with warm water. Place the soaking wet washcloth over your eyes for about three to five minutes every night. The purpose of the warm compresses is to get into the meibomian glands that line the lid to help get the oils flowing more freely. Remember that the meibomian glands make the top, oily layer of the tear film. By putting a warm compress on the lid, it is like putting butter in the microwave. You will see the clumps of oil stuck on the lid melt and flow across the front of the eye.

Lid scrubs: If you have debris on the lashes or clumps of oil stuck in the meibomian glands that line the lid, the oils will not be able to come onto the surface of the eye. Therefore, it is a good idea to use a lid scrub a minimum of once a week to cleanse the front of the eye. My favorite lid scrub is super cheap! Take a dab of baby shampoo on a washcloth and make it foamy. Then just run the washcloth across the closed eye.

Preservative-free artificial tears: If we have attempted all the aforementioned lifestyle changes and the patient is still uncomfortable, it is time to start artificial tears. Please consider that preservative-free artificial tears are not a medication, and you cannot become dependent on them. I am specifying that you use preservative-free tears that come in individual vials. I typically lean more towards these individual vials for severe dry eye cases because the preservative in traditional artificial tears can compound the patient's problems into a severe dry eye case.

The drop regimen that I typically recommend in a severe dry eye case is one drop of preservative-free artificial tear every hour on the hour for two to three full days, followed by one drop four times a day. You need so many drops for the two to three days because the entire front surface of the eye regenerates fairly rapidly, especially when well lubricated. These drops help to facilitate the production of cells that cover the front of the eye.

Part of the reason dry eye patients feel so uncomfortable is that the cells that cover the front of the eye die and are not replaced. When you use a ton of artificial tears and all of the cells are replaced, the patient feels dramatically more comfortable. After two to three days of excessive preservative-free artificial tear use, you can back down to four times a day for maintenance. My patients often ask how long they are going to have to follow the four times a day routine, and, quite frankly, I do not know. Some people can cut back on the drop use and still feel comfortable, while other people need to keep using artificial tears for some time.

Position of lids: An important part of my dry eye assessment is to take a good look at the lids and see if they are closing properly. If the patient has paralysis of the lids or has lid anatomy that prevents the lids from closing properly, the eye will be very dry. Sometimes I even ask the spouse or significant other if the patient sleeps with their eyes open. If the patient has dryness due to lid positioning, there is a wide range of treatment options ranging from surgery to thicker ointment at night. As you could probably guess, I typically try to recommend the thick ointment at night before I jump to surgery.

Medication in the form of drops: I usually try to avoid using medication if I can. However, on occasion, the patient is still significantly symptomatic despite all attempts with the medication-free route. In this case, we have many drops that we can consider, ranging from a light steroid to drops that act on the immune system to help reduce dryness. The discussion of all the forms of medication for dry eye syndrome is beyond the scope of this book. I do want to mention it so that you know that there is more advanced treatment in the case that all efforts to control the symptoms using diet and lifestyle are unsuccessful.

Procedural options: For significant dry eye, there are some easy, non-surgical medical procedures that are aimed at reducing eye dryness. For instance, the physician can put tiny stoppers in the sink holes in the corner of your eyes, like when you plug your sink. These stoppers help keep the tears around longer and can significantly reduce dry eye syndrome. They are referred to as punctal plugs.

Another procedure that is becoming more and more common is an amniotic membrane graft. This sounds super scary, but it is so easy and very effective in the case of severe dry eye. There are different types of grafts, and it is not our goal to describe each type of amniotic membrane, but the procedure is as simple as putting on a contact lens, and one to two weeks later, you feel so much better. This option is not right for everyone and is not my first line of treatment. I include these procedural options so that you know there are more advanced treatments available.

Glaucoma: You Can't Smoke Weed in Your Sleep

Before you get excited about smoking marijuana with the diagnosis of glaucoma, let's break down what glaucoma is and what we can do to control it naturally. Glaucoma is the most common cause of irreversible blindness worldwide. What makes this condition even scarier is that it is symptomless. Typically, there is no discomfort associated with glaucoma, and there is no vision loss unless the glaucoma is very advanced. Because no one can "feel" glaucoma coming on, 50 percent of those people suffering from this sight-threatening disease are undiagnosed.

I will tell you a super short story. At one of my doctor appointments to evaluate the back part of my eye, the doctors found that the pressure in my eyes had skyrocketed from the normal twelve to nearly thirty. I felt totally fine, and my vision was stable. Even though I am an eye doctor who understands that glaucoma is symptomless, I could not believe that my pressure was so high, and I told the doctor that his machine had to be broken. Being the stubborn stinker-pot that I am, I asked him to check my pressure three times with different instruments because I could not put my fingers around the fact that my pressure was elevated. The doctor patiently repeated the test and did not give me the eye roll that I certainly deserved. When I was finally convinced that the pressure was, in fact, elevated, he looked carefully at the front part of my eye only to find out that I had a form of glaucoma called angle-closure glaucoma.

Angle-closure glaucoma is a type of glaucoma that occurs because part of the eye closes off so fluid cannot drain, and the pressure builds up. One cause of angle-closure glaucoma is just having a small eyeball. Well, needless to say, I have small eyeballs, so it was no surprise that I developed this type of glaucoma.

When my physician and I determined that I, indeed, had glaucoma, I joked around with him, "Awesome, now I need to get my medical marijuana license." I knew that I would have to smoke a ton of weed all day, every day, in order to keep my pressure low enough to reduce the risk of glaucoma.

Because even marijuana would not truly fix my eye condition, we decided to do a very simple procedure where a small hole was put in the iris of the eye to relieve the pressure in the eye and virtually eliminate the risk of blindness. This is a perfect example of how nutrition, diet, and lifestyle cannot cure everything.

Quick Review of Anatomy

Just behind the front of the eye is a body of water called the anterior chamber. The anterior chamber holds water called the aqueous that provides nutrients to the front part of the eye. Where the colored part of the eye, the white of the eye, and the cornea meet is called the trabecular meshwork—this is a big fancy word for a drain line.

If this drain line is blocked or if too much fluid builds up, the pressure in the eye increases. This puts pressure on the back part of the eye, and less blood gets to the structure that connects the eye to the brain called the optic nerve. This can result in permanent loss of vision working from the outside into the central vision. This process is more complicated because there can be a slow death of the optic nerve without an increase in pressure. For that reason, it is important to turn to your eye care professional for a thorough exam annually to ensure that you do not have this blinding eye disease.

Four Most Common Types of Glaucoma

Primary open angle glaucoma: This is, by far, the most common type of glaucoma. There is typically an increase in pressure in the eye due to slowed draining of fluid in the front part of the eye, as previously described.

Angle-closure glaucoma: I was diagnosed with this form of glaucoma. This is where the drain line—located at the intersection of the cornea, white part of the eye, and the iris—becomes blocked so fluid cannot drain. If this structure becomes completely blocked, the patient may experience headaches, nausea, and vomiting.

Normal-tension glaucoma: In normal-tension glaucoma, the pressure is normal, but there is still damage to the optic nerve. For that reason, you cannot look solely at the pressure in the eye to determine if you have this potentially blinding eye disease.

Secondary glaucoma: Secondary glaucoma is glaucoma that results from something such as medication, injury, or surgery. For instance, long-term use of steroids can cause secondary glaucoma.

What Increases Someone's Risk for Developing Glaucoma?

Some of the things that put a patient at higher risk for glaucoma include the following:

Age: In general, people who are older are at higher risk of developing glaucoma. This is especially true for primary open-angle glaucoma. However, all rules are meant to be broken! I was only thirty-six when I was diagnosed with angle-closure glaucoma.

Smoking: Smoking cigarettes puts you at a much higher risk of developing glaucoma. You can pretty much assume that every condition that I mention in this book gets worse with smoking.

Family history: There is a significant increase in the risk of glaucoma when someone in the family has been diagnosed with this disease.

Race: It's always amazing to me that there is such a strong correlation between certain diseases and ethnic backgrounds. In the case of glaucoma, the risk of developing primary open angle glaucoma increases dramatically in the African American population. On the contrary, Asian Americans and Native Americans are more likely to get angle-closure glaucoma.

Medical conditions: There are many medical conditions linked to an increased risk of developing glaucoma. These conditions include diabetes, obesity, high blood pressure, cardiovascular disease, and high cholesterol.

Medications: There are several medications that can increase your risk of developing glaucoma. Antidepressants, antihistamines, steroids, and dilating drops are a few medications on this long list.

What Tests are Done to Determine If Someone Has Glaucoma?

You must understand that every doctor is different, and I cannot tell you exactly what your doctor will do during your eye exam. My goal here is to tell you some of the tests that I consider for a glaucoma workup. You can always ask your doctor about any of the tests I mention here, but you have to trust your doctor's professional opinion. These tests are not listed in any specific order.

Case history: It is important to gather demographic information, medical history, and family medical history because we need to consider the risk factors that increase the patient's glaucoma risk.

Vision/glasses prescription: Even though vision is typically unaffected in glaucoma, it is always good to check it. Obtaining the glasses prescription is also key because farsighted individuals have an increased risk of certain types of glaucoma.

Intraocular pressure: There are many ways to check the pressure inside the eyeball. Two of the most common techniques are the air puff, otherwise known as non-contact tonometry, and applanation tonometry. The gold standard is applanation tonometry. This test involves a yellow numbing drop and a probe pressing on the eye. As we discussed earlier, an increase in intraocular pressure can be linked to glaucoma.

Corneal thickness measurement (pachymetry): This is a super simple test that can either be done with a hand-held device or part of a larger machine. We care about the thickness of the cornea because if the cornea is thinner than normal, the pressure in the eye is higher than we are finding when we do the test. Likewise, if the corneal thickness is thicker than normal, the pressure is less than what we find when performing the test. The average corneal thickness measurement is around 555 micrometers.

Visual field: The visual field is a side vision test. This is one of the most boring tests in the whole world! During a visual field or perimetry test, you stick your head in a big bowl with one eye covered and push a button every time you see a light flash in your side vision. If you have ADD like Albert Einstein and me, this test is a bit of a challenge! Given that glaucoma affects the side vision first, the visual field assessment is vital in evaluating for glaucoma.

Retina/optic nerve evaluation: Obviously, it is important to look at the optic nerve because there are a number of changes in the shape and color of this structure as glaucoma progresses. When possible, photodocumentation is the best form of documentation.

Gonioscopy: During gonioscopy, the doctor puts a contact lens-like instrument onto the front part of the eye that allows the physician to look at the trabecular meshwork. The physician looks to see if the area is open or closed.

Ocular coherence tomography (OCT): This is like an ultrasound of the back part of the eye. Using this test, the doctor can evaluate the thickness of the area in and around the optic nerve. If the patient is developing glaucoma, the tissue in this area may be thinning.

Treatment

Reduce inflammation: We know that there is some "oxidative stress" associated with glaucoma. If you recall our free radical analogy from earlier, oxidative stress is when free radicals are having some serious rages, and the antibody police cannot control them. This oxidative stress wreaks havoc on the body. Although we know that this process is occurring, there is inconclusive data to support that vitamin supplementation and/or a change in diet directly lowers the pressure.

Weight loss: In the case of obesity, hypertension, and diabetes, weight loss and control of blood sugar will reduce your risk of developing glaucoma. Controlling the underlying medical condition results in better control of glaucoma.

Marijuana: I know you are excited to hear that pot really does lower the pressure in your eyes as much as 60–65 percent! That sounds like the miracle cure but hold your horses. The effects of pot are temporary, and you would need to smoke as much weed as Cheech and Chong to keep your pressure low all the time. Medical marijuana has a powerful place in treating many conditions, from Parkinson's disease to rheumatoid arthritis and pain management to fibromyalgia. As much as I would like to tell you to go smoke weed to lower your eye pressure, it just isn't the best treatment option.

Eye drops: Most forms of glaucoma are controlled with drops in the eyes. The eye doctor needs to look at the results of the tests that we talked about earlier to determine how aggressively to treat glaucoma and will come up with a treatment regimen ranging from something like one drop every night at bedtime to several drops in the morning and at night. The glaucoma doctor will want to see you on a fairly regular basis to make sure the pressure is under adequate control.

Surgery: Depending on the type of glaucoma and the severity of the damage, the physician may opt to do surgery as a first-line treatment. Surgery, however, is not typically the first line of treatment for the most common types of glaucoma. Glaucoma surgery may be as simple as poking holes in the drain line called the trabecular meshwork to help it drain better and as complex as putting in an artificial plastic drain to help get the fluid out of the front of the eye.

Diabetes, Obesity, and Hypertension: The Three Stooges

Comorbidity and Eye Disease

Diabetes, hypertension, and obesity are kind of like Moe, Larry, and Curly of The Three Stooges. They are damaging as individuals, but when they are all in the same room, they are disastrous. Pretty much everyone reading this book has a friend or family member with diabetes. Diabetes is oftentimes coupled with hypertension or obesity. In the medical world, this is called comorbidity, something that also—"*co-*"—can lead to death—"*-morbidity.*" Your next question may be, why are we so concerned about all of these medical conditions, isn't this supposed to be an eye book? You should get the pattern by now that the eye is the window to the body, and with its tiny, fragile blood vessels, these diseases show up in the eye first.

I am going to tell you about the day that I saved a patient's life. A very sweet 55-year-old heavy-set lady came to my office for a routine eye exam because she said her contacts were not working anymore. She noticed it most when working on the computer and watching television. She was sure that a subtle change in her contact lens script would fix the problem. I checked this lady's vision, and the best glasses in the world were not going to help her see. I would go so far as to say that this lady would not have passed her driver's vision test even with the best pair of glasses man could buy.

My heart was dropping for her as I was conducting the eye exam because I knew we were headed down a tough road. When we discussed her medical history, she told me that her blood pressure was high in the past and that she had it under control with medication. I went on to check her blood pressure, and it was 240/160 mmHg! I could not believe my eyes. I checked it again, and it was super elevated. I was surprised the lady was alive with blood pressure that high. I immediately called 911, beaconing an ambulance to take her to the emergency room—*STAT*.

While we waited for the paramedic to arrive, I looked at the back of her eye because I was concerned about what was going on back there. Not to my surprise, hypertension had done considerable damage to the back of her eye. The only thing that gave me comfort at this point was that I knew we could give her some vision back by helping her get her blood pressure under control.

My patient requested that I call her daughter to explain the situation and ensure that she had company at the hospital. I kept in contact with this lady and her daughter for a number of days as she worked her way from the emergency room to the ICU and eventually was on her way to recovery. Within a day, I got the sweetest phone call from her daughter! I could see the tears in her eyes and hear the lump in her throat as she told me that the emergency room doctors told her mother would have been dead within a week if not for her visit to the eye doctor.

This is just one example of how important it is to get your yearly comprehensive eye exam because diseases like diabetes and high blood pressure show up in the eye first. Luckily, for those of you who have not been to the eye doctor lately, there are some great options out there to help the doctor see 99 percent of the back part of your eye without eye drops using a widefield retina camera. This technology has revolutionized the way we practice!

Diabetes

Before we get into our discussion of eye diseases, let's take a step back and review what diabetes is and its effect on the eye. My purpose in explaining the details here is to help you understand what causes diabetes to understand the natural treatment options.

When we get hungry, we eat. We need food to give us energy. The way you get energy from the food is pretty interesting. Food enters your mouth and works its way into your tummy. There is an organ about six inches long and located behind the stomach that affects the fate of the food you just ate. This organ is called the pancreas, and it is connected to your digestive tract via a tiny tube called a duct. The mighty pancreas makes a hormone called insulin that it sends to the digestive tract via this tube. Insulin is like the dinner bell for the body. It tells the cells that the food has arrived and it's time to eat. The cells open their little cellular mouths and eat the glucose to get their energy.

Carbohydrates get such a bad reputation! I think it's important to talk about what this curse word in the dieter's vocabulary really means. Carbohydrates are like our body's gasoline. Your car cannot run without gas unless it is electric. Well, your body cannot survive without carbohydrates. Carbohydrates are sugars and starches that are broken down to glucose. Glucose is used by the tiny cells in our body to do literally everything that it needs to do. Without glucose, we would die.

It does not take much for this whole system to go to hell in a handbasket. First of all, on occasion, an autoimmune problem can cause damage to the parts of the pancreas that makes insulin, and absolutely no insulin is produced. This is a huge problem, and it is called type 1 diabetes. The second main problem to talk about is called type 2 diabetes. This is when the pancreas releases less insulin, or the body does not react to the insulin that is released. The body ignoring the insulin released is called insulin resistance. Some of the main things that cause type 2 diabetes are age, increased belly fat, smoking, insufficient exercise, and poor sleep quality; of course, always consider family history.

You are probably wondering what effect all of this stuff with diabetes really has on the body. Well, funny, you should ask! The eye is one of the first organs to be affected by diabetes. The tiny blood vessels in the eye are very fragile, and the series of events that I just described makes the blood vessels weak and leaky. As a result, we often find blood vessel bleeds, and leakage in the eye before the patient even knows that they have diabetes. Some of the things that we see as eye care physicians in a diabetic patient are blood spots on the back part of the eye, thickening of the best central vision area in the back part of the eye, leakage from blood vessels, and dramatic changes in the eyeglass prescription.

Hypertension

Simply put, hypertension is when the blood pressure is too high, but what is scary about hypertension is it is symptomless; it is "the silent killer." The reason why this is a problem is because you can get all sorts of other problems like heart failure, kidney failure, and strokes. However, the effect of hypertension that we are most concerned about for the purpose of this book is damage to the eye called retinopathy.

I will give you a super-fast lecture on assessing blood pressure. Although the determination of whether or not you have high blood pressure should, ultimately, be made by your physician, the normal reading is 120/80 mmHg. The first number is your systolic reading, and the second number is your diastolic reading. High blood pressure is considered anything over 130 mmHg on the systolic or anything over 80 on the diastolic. Your doctor may ask you to measure your blood pressure at different times of the day at home. The goal here is two-fold. First of all, we can see if your blood pressure fluctuates at different times of the day. Secondly, we can see if you have higher blood pressure in the doctor's office, a condition known as white coat syndrome.

Let's talk about what raises your risk of getting high blood pressure. Social habits of smoking, drinking alcohol, and a lack of exercise certainly contribute to your risk. However, some of the biggest risk factors for the development of high blood pressure are being diabetic and overweight.

Why is this disease so critical for us to discuss? Almost 50 percent of American adults have hypertension, and most of these people do not have their hypertension under control. Uncontrolled hypertension can result in changes to the back part of the eye. This is hypertensive retinopathy. The range of damage to the eye due to high blood pressure can range from very mild to blinding. In mild hypertensive retinopathy, we may find changes to the shape of the blood vessels. In moderate hypertensive retinopathy, we can find blood spots or white patches on the back part of the eye that look like cotton or wool, namely, cotton wool spots. When the high blood pressure is severe, the nerve that connects the eye to the brain gets swollen, and it looks like it is popping out of the back part of the eye. This is what I saw in the lady that I sent to the emergency room.

Diabetes and Obesity

We talk about diabetes and obesity together because they usually go hand in hand. An obese individual takes more energy to move oftentimes feels lethargic. This person may turn to food for energy. With food consumption, insulin is released by the pancreas. This results in more and more glucose in our blood. Our bodies can only use so much glucose for energy, so any unused glucose is stored as fat. The stored fat makes the person more sluggish. It is a vicious cycle continuously making the person more overweight and more tired. Eventually, the pancreas checks out and says it's going on a vacation because it is overworked and underpaid. The body decides to boycott work along with the pancreas and starts to ignore the insulin. This compounds the problem, and you end up with type 2 diabetes.

What makes obesity even more difficult to deal with is the stigma that goes along with being overweight. As a physician, it is not difficult for me to discuss social history, including smoking and drinking habits, with my patients. I let the patients know that I am not judgey, but I need to know if they are smoking because it raises risks of several diseases. It is much more difficult to discuss weight with my patients as it can raise lots of emotions. Most patients do not look to the eye doctor for weight counseling, but it plays a big part in the assessment of the eye.

How do we really define obesity? I hate technical terms, but you need to understand one basic term, Body Mass Index (BMI). Body Mass Index takes into account two things, your height and weight. When you put these numbers into the magical BMI calculator, you come up with a numerical value of your amount of body fat. You are looking for this number to be anywhere from 18–24. Although being a little on the overweight side sounds like no big deal, the list of problems associated with obesity is lengthy. Here are a few, just to give you an idea:

- Increased risk of stroke: Strokes can even occur in the eye!
- Increased risk of heart attack
- Sleep apnea: Another disease that can cause an eye problem is called floppy eyelid syndrome.
- Increased risk of diabetes: We already talked about how diabetes can affect the eye.
- Kidney and liver failure
- Depression

The Eye Exam

The blood vessels in the retina are super fragile, and the first part of the eye to be affected by diabetes, high blood pressure, and obesity. There is a plethora of tests that can be used to assess the back part of the eye thoroughly. The gold standard retina evaluation will always be dilation when the doctor puts drops in the eye to make the pupil super large then looks in using super bright lights. This can be super uncomfortable and does not allow you to track changes of practically every square inch of your eye. For that reason, brilliant scientific minds developed the widefield retina camera, which provides a great option to see almost every square inch of your and photo-document the results to simplify the doctor's ability to changes year after year.

Eye doctors can also see a cross-section of the back part of the eye like an ultrasound called an ocular coherence tomography (OCT). This machine gives more detail about damage to the most vulnerable parts of the eye, allowing early detection of diabetes in the eye. Even more advanced testing is called fluorescein angiography, which involves shooting dye in your arm and IV and evaluating how the dye moves through the blood vessels in your eye.

Treatment

First and foremost, it is important to have an early diagnosis of these conditions. Annual evaluations with your primary care doctor and eye care provider are a must. Catching these diseases early makes the treatment much more manageable.

More and more doctors are turning to diet and lifestyle as a first-line treatment for these conditions. I bet you are as sick of hearing about diet and lifestyle as you are hearing about coronavirus. Changing your diet and modifying your lifestyle sounds like torcher, right? I get it. I have been there. Take a deep breath, and let's talk about some simple changes that you may be able to make to get yourself back on track. We are going to go into much more detail about each of these points in the *Beyond Carrots* Plan, so this is just a teaser.

1. I know you don't want to hear this, but thirty minutes of exercise five days a week will work wonders. I promise you will be excited to exercise after covering it further in one of the following chapters.
2. Small changes to diet go a long way. Pay attention to the amount of sugar you put into your body. If you can cut out all soda and processed foods, you will be on your way to reducing weight.
3. Relaxation is key. Stress can raise blood pressure and increase food consumption. This drives blood sugar through the roof and raises the risk of diabetes. The excess sugar in the blood is stored as fat which raises BMI and causes obesity.
4. Stop smoking. I am starting to sound like my mother with the number of times I repeat myself on the smoking thing.
5. Moderate alcohol consumption. If I can do moderate alcohol con-

sumption, you can too. Once again, I find myself sounding like my mother!

Uveitis: A Big Word for Inflammation

This section is near and dear to my heart because my diagnosis was associated with uveitis. This particular eye disease is very scary because you could be on the road to blindness and not even know it. Unlike cataracts, glaucoma, and macular degeneration, very few people have even heard of uveitis. If I went around and asked my patients if they had heard of "uveitis," I would say that 96 percent of them would say they do not know this term. However, uveitis is one of the world's leading causes of blindness. It has been estimated that 10–15 percent of the people who are severely visually handicapped can attribute their vision loss to uveitis. My goal is to help educate you on what to look for to help bring awareness to the underdog, uveitis.

My condition, known as idiopathic retinal vasculitis, is incredibly rare and most commonly affects healthy females between thirty and forty years old. These women typically have an otherwise clean bill of health. The patient is generally made aware that they have the disease only when they are handicapped due to their vision loss. This is a scary condition! I was lucky because I made it to the doctor just in the nick of time. If I had waited as few as a couple of months, I would be irreversibly blind. What is equally important to note is that this is all controllable if caught early enough and managed properly.

Uveitis symptoms may be as subtle as a floater. However, other cases of uveitis may be quite bothersome, and the patient may experience redness, significant discomfort, pain, blurred vision, and headaches. This is part of why when I get a phone call to my office with a patient telling me that they just have a little pink eye, I always ask to evaluate the patient in person. I need to closely examine all patients for any of the signs of uveitis before I dismiss the patient as simple conjunctivitis.

What is Uveitis Anyway?

Any condition that ends with the four letters I-T-I-S is inflammatory in nature. In the case of uveitis, there is inflammation of the uvea. What the heck is the uvea? The uvea is the part of the eye that includes three main structures. You may want to go back to that handy-dandy drawing of the eye as we talk about these structures.

The first structure of the uvea is the iris. This is the colored part of the eye. When you talk about someone having blue, green, hazel, or brown eyes, you are describing the iris. The second part of the uvea is the choroid. The choroid is a part of the retina that is like a big bunch of blood vessels that bring blood to the retina. Remember that the retina is the back part of the eye where light focuses. The third structure of the uvea is the ciliary body which includes the ciliary muscle. The ciliary body causes the lens of your eye to adjust its focus so that you can see. Additionally, the ciliary body makes the water that fills the front part of the eye.

To make things more complicated, there are four types of uveitis. Being that this is not a medical textbook, I am going to simplify this for you.

- **Anterior uveitis:** inflammation of the uvea that affects the front part of the eye, including the iris and ciliary body.
- **Intermediate uveitis:** inflammation of the middle structures of the eye, including the big ball of jelly in the back part of the eye and the peripheral retina.
- **Posterior uveitis:** inflammation of the choroid, the big meshwork of blood vessels that carry vital nutrients to the retina.
- **Panuveitis:** Everything in the front, middle, and back parts of the eye is inflamed. Symptoms associated with anterior uveitis are redness, pain, discomfort, and headaches.

What Causes Uveitis?

The most common causes of uveitis are autoimmune diseases, infections, and inflammatory diseases. Some of the most common autoimmune diseases that are linked to uveitis are rheumatoid arthritis, ankylosing spondylitis, and sarcoidosis. An example of an infection that can cause uveitis is herpes simplex, Lyme disease, and syphilis. Some of the inflammatory diseases that can cause uveitis are Crohn's disease and ulcerative colitis.

How Can I Get Tested for Uveitis?

The best thing to do to be sure that you do not have uveitis is to get a full eye exam every year with a complete evaluation of the retina. I believe every single patient should have widefield photodocumentation of the back part of the eye as part of the eye exam. Widefield photos are different than standard photos as they help the doctor see the majority of the back part of the eye and keep that photo on file for review year after year. I am partial to this particular type of photodocumentation because this is the test that I was a guinea pig for at the conference when I found the retina blood spots in my eyes. If not for this camera, I would be blind right now.

If the doctor sees an abnormality when doing the widefield retina photo, the doctor will decide whether or not to refer you to a specialist for further evaluation. When you go to a specialist, more information can be gathered about uveitis by doing a test where the physician shoots dye in the arm and watches it as it flows through the blood vessels. This test is fluorescein angiography. The specialist may also want to do an OCT, which is like an ultrasound of your eye. The OCT shows the physician what is going on with every layer of the back part of the eye and tells the doctor the thickness of these structures.

If it is determined that you have uveitis, the doctor may opt to order a plethora of additional tests, including inflammatory marker blood workup, chest X-Ray, tuberculosis testing, and Lyme disease testing. The full scope of tests included in a uveitis workup is way beyond the scope of this book. Suffice to say, there are a ton of things that need to be ruled out before a diagnosis is made.

Traditional Treatment for Uveitis

I know all too much about the traditional treatment for uveitis because I experienced this disease firsthand. The main goal when treating uveitis is to reduce inflammation, eliminate pain, and prevent vision loss.

Steroids, either topical or oral, are sometimes used to control the inflammation. When the inflammation is reduced, there is less pain. The problem with steroids is that extended steroid use can cause a whole slew of medical conditions ranging from osteoporosis and diabetes to cataracts and glaucoma. Steroids are not a practical long-term solution for uveitis. To make matters worse, abruptly stopping steroids can cause the inflammatory condition to come back with a vengeance. For that reason, a gradual reduction of the amount of steroids is recommended.

Another possible treatment of uveitis is immunosuppressive therapy with drugs such as methotrexate and daclizumab. The list of side effects for these drugs is extensive as they can damage nearly every organ of your body, from your liver to your kidney, and they can increase the risk of cancer.

On occasion, injections and laser surgery are necessary for treating uveitis. The injection is done in an attempt to control the inflammation. On the other hand, laser surgery is done to kill off part of the retina that is already dead so that no new blood vessels form. The eye creates new blood vessels in areas where there is no blood flow as a last-ditch effort to get blood to this area of the eye. Unfortunately, these new blood vessels are weak and break easily, potentially causing significant vision loss. After laser surgery to the retina, the eye forfeits its fight and will not try to make new blood vessels.

How I Got My Condition to Take a Hike

I was treated with laser surgery and oral steroids for almost six months when I switched to immunosuppressive therapy. I drew the line here and started to take matters into my own hands. I developed a treatment protocol to treat my inflammatory condition that started with healing my gut. The gut? Yup. You heard me right. I realized that by fixing up my tummy, I would help to reverse the eye problem. It was my hope that I would be able to avoid all treatment. It turns out my inclination was correct.

Through my research, I determined that there was a direct connection between the gut and the eye, similar to the connection that the gut has with the brain. You may or may not realize that bacteria are living all over your body. Every square inch of your body is covered with creepy crawlies. Our natural first reaction is ICK!

But, on second thought, you would not be alive without these bacteria. The gut has more bacteria than other parts of the body. Something like 100 trillion bacteria live in the gut. When these bacteria are not balanced, it triggers an immune response in the brain and in the eye. The body thinks that there is an intruder and is trying to kill it by activating its killer cells. This system goes south quickly when the body gets confused and starts attacking its own cells instead of intruder cells because the cells look so similar. This is called an autoimmune response.

By healing the gut and keeping the good bacteria around, we minimize this immune reaction and control the inflammation. This is a perfect segue to our next chapter, where we talk about specifically what we need to do to heal the gut.

Chapter 4:
What to Eat and What to Avoid

Gut Health-Your First Line of Defense

I cannot overemphasize how important it is to understand that your eyes are connected to your body. There is a reason why we ask a million and one questions about your health history when you come in for an eye exam. I will give you an example that many people can relate to. If you stay up partying till 4:00 a.m. doing a bar crawl in Fort Lauderdale, your eyes will be bloodshot, and your lids may be swollen in the morning.

Here's another example. Have you ever noticed what happens to your eyes when you see a scary scene in a movie? If you were to video your eyes as you get scared, you would see your eyes open wider and your pupils dilate. My point here is that your mind, your body, and your eyes are all connected.

Taking that point one step further, your brain and your gut also communicate with one another. The word "gut" has become popular in the health arena over the past five to ten years. You can think of the gut as everything from your mouth to your butt. How are the two connected? Have you ever ordered out a heavy lunch and noticed that you want to crash afterward? How about the good old adage, "I got so scared, I just about s--- my pants?"

Emotions have an effect on bowel movements. Anyone with irritable bowel syndrome can attest to the fact that stress has a direct effect on their tummy condition. The connection between the brain and digestion won Ivan Pavlov a Nobel Prize in 1904. Pavlov showed that when food was presented to a dog, saliva and digestive enzymes were released.

Now that we know that that the eyes are connected to the body and that the brain is connected to the gut, let's talk about what happens in the gut. The gut is your first line of defense between you and the outside world. You can think of your gut as a big tube extending from your mouth to your anus filled with mucus, bacteria, and chemicals that break down food. We will call this tube the digestive tract. The digestive tract has two main purposes. The first, most obvious, function is to break down food and absorb the nutrients to fuel the body. An equally important role of this tube is to protect our bodies from the outside world. Even if you scrub your apples with soap and water, soak your spinach in vinegar water, and eat the highest-grade organic meat, you still ingest bad things that can damage your body if they make their way through the walls of the digestive tract.

We are all covered in bacteria! Don't go running to your shower; it is not going to help. It has been estimated that there are one trillion bacteria all over your skin. Equally as impressive is the fact that there are almost one hundred times more bacteria in the gut than on the skin, amounting to almost one hundred trillion bacteria in your gut! It may seem counterintuitive, but it is the bacteria in the digestive tract that help to protect our bodies. In a symbiotic relationship, the bacteria that live in the gut and the body benefit from one another. Symbiotic relationships are often found in nature. For example, a flower provides a bee with nectar, and the bee aids in spreading pollen and fertilization of the plant. Similarly, the bacteria have a safe place to live on the body, and the little buggers keep the bad stuff out.

However, not all bacteria are helpful to our bodies. Some bacteria that enter the digestive tract are quite damaging. When there are more bad bacteria than good bacteria, the symbiotic relationship that we talked about earlier is disrupted. This is called gut dysbiosis. Now that you understand what symbiosis means, you can better understand how the term gut dysbiosis was derived. I want to focus on two things that can happen with gut dysbiosis that can be thought of as confusion in our bodies' armies and broken guard gates.

When the bad bacteria overpopulate the gut, and we have gut dysbiosis, the body is alerted. It goes into attack mode to get the bacteria out of its first line of defense area ASAP. The body sends its army out to kill the bacteria. The armies of our bodies gets geared up and has a big meeting where they discuss what the targeted bacteria looks like.

For discussion's sake, let's say that the army says that the invaders are wearing a Chicago Cubs t-shirt. After the meeting, the army sets out to kill all invaders wearing a Chicago Cubs t-shirt. Well, unfortunately, some of the army members get confused and start attacking when they see a Chicago Bears t-shirt. OOPS! The cells with a Chicago Bears t-shirt happen to be a part of the person's own body. This army made a mistake, and the body is now attacking itself. This is an autoimmune reaction.

The second problem that I want to talk about relating to gut dysbiosis is regarding the guard gates in our gut. We need to understand that there are gates all over our digestive tract. When there is gut dysbiosis, and bad bacteria overtake the gut, the bacteria release a chemical that breaks the chain keeping the drawbridges pulled up. When the drawbridge is down, our castle protection is destroyed, and the first line of defense is defeated. Any invader can stomp right on into our bodies and destroy anything and everything in its path. When the body tries to kill the invader, the autoimmune response is exacerbated. This problem has been labeled by the health and fitness world as leaky gut syndrome.

What Came First, the Chicken or the Egg?

The list of medical conditions linked to gut dysbiosis is overwhelming. Diabetes, hypertension, obesity, ADD/ADHD, rheumatoid arthritis, celiac disease, and multiple sclerosis, to name a few. As high as 70 percent of autism cases have problems with the gut. Symptoms such as brain fog, fatigue, disrupted complexion, headaches, and depression have been linked to gut dysbiosis.

What came first, the chicken (the disease) or the egg (gut dysbiosis)? This is a topic of debate among functional medicine physicians and some skeptics. I am not going to get in the middle of that debate. However, fixing our gut's drawbridges and replenishing the good bacteria will reverse medical conditions and reduce the aforementioned symptoms related to gut dysbiosis.

Remind Me Again Why We are Talking about The Gut in an Eye Book? Bottom Line Points Regarding Gut Health:

- The gut and the eyes are connected, so when the good and bad bacteria in the gut are out of balance, the eyes are affected.
- Uveitis: I have to mention this one first because this is the one I conquered through diet and nutrition. My plan to repair my eyes started with fixing my gut.
- Dry eye/Sjogren's Syndrome: Sjogren's Syndrome is an autoimmune

disease that affects the eyes, causing many symptoms, including dry eyes and dry mouth. Curing the gut will help reverse these diseases.
- Diabetes and obesity: Pretty much anyone with diabetes and obesity has some gut dysbiosis.
- Hypertension: You will often find more bad bacteria in the gut with a patient who has hypertension and other cardiovascular diseases.
- Age-Related Macular Degeneration: Fixing the gut will reduce the risk of developing macular degeneration.

Gut Repair

Popular media has made the "Four Rs of Gut Repair" almost cliche. If you have heard about leaky gut syndrome, then you have probably heard of the Four Rs of Gut Repair. As overdone as it may seem, these Four Rs actually work! The CliffNotes version of the Four Rs of Gut Repair is to eat whole foods, eliminate toxins, take probiotics, and fix the guard gates. I mean, you cannot go wrong doing that? No wonder why it works. Let's break it down so that you understand what really goes into this process.

Remove: Remove bad things from your diet and surroundings. There are a number of foods that cause inflammation of the gut lining and can irritate your gut. For example, you may have heard about the notorious gluten. There is a school of thought that gluten essentially breaks the chain that holds the draw bridges of our gut up. According to this philosophy, when we eat gluten, our gut goes to hell in a handbasket. Perhaps equally as damaging is dairy. Your body recognizes dairy as foreign and instantly goes into attack mode. Eggs, dairy, corn, soy, sugar, alcohol, and caffeine are also some of the big ones.

Medicines that are meant to help our bodies can have a detrimental effect on the gut. For instance, we may take antibiotics to kill a bacterial infection. Unfortunately, these antibiotics also kill the good bacteria in our gut, throwing off the balance between good and bad bacteria and throwing the body into gut dysbiosis.

Toxins are another big culprit in the destruction of the gut. Toxins are all over us and can range in their presentation from pesticides in foods and sulfates in wines to chemicals used in facial products or cleaning supplies. Even air can have toxins such as toxic mold.

Stress and gut dysbiosis also go hand in hand. When you are stressed, your brain communicates with the gut, and the stress hormones throw the gut into disarray.

Replace: When the bad bacteria overpopulate and the walls of the gut get inflamed, the enzymes that are normally around to digest food are thrown out of kilter. The second "R" refers to the process of replacing enzymes that are necessary for proper food digestion so that you can extract the vital nutrients from the whole foods you are eating. Without these enzymes around, food goes undigested right through your body. As a result, you eat but don't feel nourished, so you feel tired and end up trying to eat more to get the nutrition that you are lacking. By replacing the digestive enzymes, you break down food better and get the nutrition you need so you feel more energized without overeating.

Reinoculated: This one is pretty obvious. You need to restore the good bacteria. This is where probiotics come into play.

Repair: This is where the drawbridges are repaired, and the inflammation in the gut lining is calmed. One of the best ways to repair the drawbridge is by eating prebiotics. Prebiotics are fibrous food that serves as food for the good bacteria in our gut. The good bacteria in our gut LOVE kale and spinach. Other high-fiber foods are artichokes and beets. Although nuts and beans are also high fiber, I would advise avoiding them initially because they can cause inflammation. Other foods that are fantastic for gut repair are bone broth and collagen. You can think of these foods as the rebuilders of our gut wall. Omega-3 fatty acids are a must here because they help reduce the inflammation in the gut and repair the lining. Lastly, vitamins A, C, E, and D are great for gut repair as they are my favorite antioxidant vitamins.

Gut Repair To-Do List

1. Eliminate any food that can cause inflammation, including the following: gluten, dairy, corn, soy, legumes, nightshades, nuts, alcohol, and caffeine.
2. Do your best to minimize toxins from your environment: buy organic vegetables and meat, use filtered water, minimize plastic container use, use an air filter when able, start transitioning to beauty and cleaning products that are non-toxic.
3. You cannot eliminate stress completely, but you can change the way you approach stressors. Consider stress management techniques

discussed in this book.
4. Discuss the damaging effects that some medicines can have on your gut and be sure to take probiotics when medication is unavoidable.
5. Consider taking a digestive enzyme supplement. You may not have a fortune to spend on supplements, so I would advise getting one that is within your budget. Anything you take here is better than nothing.
6. Start taking probiotics immediately. Look for a minimum of 50 billion CFU (colony-forming units). Again, I don't want you to go out and break the bank or decide not to take a probiotic because it costs more than you want to spend but try to get close to 50 billion CFU if you can.
7. Load up on foods rich in prebiotics that are high in fiber. Consider artichokes, carrots, apples, and pears.
8. Drink bone broth and take collagen supplementation daily. This is like a massage for your gut. Your tummy will love you for it.
9. Take 2–4 grams of fish oil daily.
10. Ensure that your multivitamin contains adequate A, C, and E vitamins.
11. Consider supplementing with vitamin D.

Gluten: I Don't Have Celiac Disease, so I Can Skip This Chapter ... Wrong!

Let's talk about how bad of a reputation gluten has gotten. In the past decade, books, television shows, and radio talk show hosts have made the general population aware of the potential problems that gluten can have on our health. This has resulted in a health food trend away from gluten. I would go so far as to say that some people feel as if they are consuming poison when the label does not indicate that the product is gluten-free. Needless to say, food manufacturers are profiting as they picked up on the desire for people to be free of this perceived food contaminant. People are willing to shell out sometimes up to double the price on an item in an attempt to be gluten-free.

When you think of gluten, what do you think of? Pizza, pasta, bread? Yummy! Interestingly, if you looked hard enough, you could find gluten in products ranging from beauty supplies to vitamin supplements. Even frozen vegetables covered in sauce can have gluten in the sauce. So, people think they are healthy by taking vitamins and eating vegetables only to find out that they are also consuming gluten.

The gluten-free craze can be related to many other popular food crazes. If you are old enough to remember growing up in the '60s, milk was considered an absolute essential in every young person's diet. More recently, there has been some skepticism regarding the consumption of dairy in children. How about the good old food pyramid? When I was growing up, I learned about the food pyramid as the only way to determine if you had a balanced diet. That idea is obsolete.

My negative tone regarding media hype and overpriced food labels is not to be confused with the idea that gluten is A-okay and completely harmless. To be honest with you, I do not know for sure. Yes, I said it; I do not know. There is still so much research to do on this topic, and the existing research is difficult to interpret. Even experts on gluten have been slightly wishy-washy in their opinion about the effects that gluten can have on the body. My goal here is to give you as much unbiased information as possible about gluten and give you the tools to make decisions for yourself. I will provide as much up-to-date data as possible, given the research available at this time.

What is Gluten? Why is It a Problem?

Gluten is a protein most commonly found in grains, barley, rye, and wheat. *Gluten* is Latin for the word "glue." It got its name because when gluten and water combine, they make a sticky substance, which helps hold foods together. The two main proteins that make up gluten are glutenin and gliadin.

One of the big problems with gluten is that one of its proteins, gliadin, looks a lot like the walls of the gut and can be easily confused by our immune system. So, when our immune system tries to deal with gliadin, it attacks our gut walls, which can cause inflammation. Therefore, gliadin is responsible for many of the problems associated with gluten. Another big problem with gluten is that it increases the release of a protein called zonulin. Some experts believe that zonulin opens holes in our gut, allowing junk to leak into our bodies, causing the autoimmune reaction I discussed earlier.

Classifications of People with Gluten Problems

Current research has divided people with gluten problems into three main groups: celiac disease, allergy to wheat, and non-celiac gluten sensitivity. In celiac disease, gluten is a real problem. For a patient with celiac disease, even a tiny bit of gluten will activate an immune reaction, and they will get inflammation all over the body. However, celiac disease only affects about one percent of people. In the case of celiac disease, there are tests that can be done to confirm the diagnosis. The tests can be as simple as a blood test and as elaborate as a small intestine biopsy. I can tell you with great confidence, if you have celiac disease, you should avoid gluten. Symptoms associated with celiac disease are bloating, abdominal pain, fatigue, headache, diarrhea, gassy feeling, and anxiety.

Wheat allergy is the second main group of people who can be affected by gluten. This group is pretty self-explanatory, as the name says it all. Blood tests show that the body has made antibodies to wheat and gliadin. As a brief recap of our antibody discussion, antibodies are around when the body is trying to attack something. Because there are antibodies to wheat and gliadin in the bloodwork, it is obvious that the body is in the body, and the body is in attack mode. When the body is in attack mode, you can get widespread inflammation. An allergy to wheat is usually clear-cut and can be detected early. Wheat allergy is present in at very most nine percent of our population. Wheat allergy can have similar effects on our bodies as any other type of allergy to food. You may see symptoms as severe swelling, hives, difficulty breathing, or as mild as an itch, nausea, vomiting, or diarrhea. The good thing about wheat allergy is that you can test for it and get a clear-cut answer as to whether or not this is your problem.

The last classification of people with gluten problems is called non-celiac gluten sensitivity (NCGS). Unlike celiac disease and wheat allergy, the tests cannot definitively diagnose people in this category. It is not like you can do a blood test and look for antibodies or look at the genetic make-up of an individual to determine if they are considered non-celiac gluten sensitive. This diagnosis is really a diagnosis that is made based on self-reported symptoms. Symptoms associated with NCGS mirror those of celiac disease. The general suggestion is that if you think you have NCGS, eliminate gluten from your diet, and if you feel better, then you have your diagnosis.

It is important to mention a couple of points regarding NCGS. First of all, there is a great deal of overlap in the symptoms associated with irritable bowel syndrome (IBS) and gluten sensitivity. IBS is a problem with the digestive tract that has been linked to stress, an overactive immune system, and various food triggers. Anyone with IBS can tell you that when you get a flair-up of IBS, you get bloating, abdominal pain, cramping, gas, and diarrhea. This list should sound familiar because it is pretty much the same as the list of celiac disease symptoms. Like NCGS, IBS is diagnosed when the doctor has done every other test in the world and cannot find anything wrong. In medicine, we call this a diagnosis of exclusion.

To make things even more confusing, we add FODMAPs. FODMAPs stands for "fermentable, oglio-, di-, monosaccharides, and polyols." These are carbohydrates often found in wheat but can also be found in fruits and vegetables ranging from artichokes and cabbage to brussels sprouts and onions. Some people have difficulties digesting these carbohydrates, and this can trigger the same list of symptoms: bloating, abdominal pain, cramping, gas, and diarrhea. FODMAPs are confusing because they are often in food that contains gluten, so we cannot be positive whether it is the FODMAPs that are causing the problem or the gluten. When a select group of people eliminates the foods containing this carbohydrate from their diet, they feel better. Eliminating FODMAPs from your diet is very complicated because many of the foods that contain this carbohydrate are part of a balanced diet, so consult a dietician if you think it could be right for you.

Another Situation That Begs the Question about the Chicken or the Egg

I am going to tell you a secret, NCGS is overwhelmingly accompanied by other autoimmune problems in the body. Problems such as rheumatoid arthritis, psoriasis, thyroid problems almost always have NCGS. Remember that in autoimmune diseases, the body attacks itself. So, putting two and two together, when you have NCGS, your entire body is in attack mode.

This raises the question of whether the gluten caused the autoimmune disease or the autoimmune disease caused the gluten sensitivity? In the case that gluten caused the autoimmune disease, the argument may be that gluten destroyed the gut, causing all sorts of bad stuff to leak out into our bodies and putting the body into attack mode. When the autoimmune disease causes gluten sensitivity, the entire body, including the gut, is inflamed. This causes an over-response to the components of gluten and a devastating effect on the body. Interestingly, both of these scenarios benefit from a gluten-free diet. My point here is that there is undoubtedly a connection between autoimmune disease and gluten sensitivity, even though the causative relationship is difficult to determine.

My Suggestion for You

My suggestion on how to handle gluten is really quite simple. If you think you are gluten sensitive, first and foremost, determine if you have celiac disease or a wheat allergy. If you have celiac disease or a wheat allergy, avoid gluten. If you do not have either of these problems but think you have gluten sensitivity, eliminate gluten from your diet and see how you feel. If you feel better, great! Stick with your gluten-free diet. If you don't feel better, investigate further. If you decide to go gluten-free, be sure to supplement with probiotics because you still need to ensure that you try to keep building up those good bacteria in your gut.

Furthermore, if you have an autoimmune disease, I can almost guarantee that you have some level of gut dysbiosis. We covered that in the last chapter. If you have gut dysbiosis, I can almost guarantee you have some level of gluten sensitivity. They all kind of go hand in hand. If you have an active autoimmune disease, avoid gluten at all costs until you get your autoimmune disease under control. Depending on how severe your condition is, it may take anywhere from thirty days to over a year. Refraining from gluten during this time is recommended. Now, it is nearly impossible to be completely gluten-free because gluten is nearly everywhere but doing your best to avoid gluten is a good idea if you have an active autoimmune condition.

One of the challenges in being gluten-free is that the gluten-free option is not always the healthy option. I will give you an example. Let's say that you have two dinner options. One option is a frozen pizza that is labeled as gluten-free with cheese and pepperoni. The other option is a beef barley soup with carrots, onions, and celery. Remember that barley has gluten, so this beef barley soup contains gluten. Which is the better dinner option? Even though the gluten-free pizza may be toxic to a person with celiac disease or wheat allergy, the added sugar and reduced nutritional value make it the less nutrient-dense option of the two. Gluten-free foods have added sugar and reduced nutritional value, giving the consumer a false sense of security around their food choices. I would encourage you to focus on eating more whole foods that are not processed and steer away from gluten when possible.

Where Can You Find Gluten?

We already talked about this, but I wanted to give you a quick reference list of some of the most common sources of gluten:

- Bread
- Rye
- Oats
- Barley
- Beer
- Wine
- Crackers
- Spices
- Pasta sauces
- Pasta
- Rice
- Salad dressings
- Soy sauce
- Condiments
- Pickles
- Couscous
- Medications
- Beauty products

In summary, there is clearly a link between gluten and autoimmune disease. I would recommend sticking to whole foods and avoiding anything that is processed, and you will be on the right track. When considering processed foods, the gluten-free option is not necessarily the more nutritious option. I would recommend doing everything in your power to control stress in your life as there is clearly a link between stress, the immune system, and gluten sensitivity.

But I Thought Tomatoes, Bell Peppers, and Zucchini were Vegetables?

No good discussion about food and eye health would be complete without a talk about tomatoes and the nightshade family of fruits. Now, this is a slightly controversial topic, and I honestly considered skipping this topic completely, but I could not do that to my readers. Here is the thing: tomatoes, bell peppers, zucchini, potatoes, and even herbs like cayenne pepper and chili pepper belong to an entire family of plants called *Solanaceae*, more commonly known as nightshades. Nightshades are an interesting bunch because the health benefits of the fruits of these plants are endless. However, when chemicals in these plants are consumed in very concentrated amounts, they can be quite toxic and possibly even fatal. That being said, it's nearly impossible to ingest so many tomatoes, zucchini, tomatoes, or any other nightshades that you actually die.

On a more practical note, some people cannot tolerate nightshades in their diet. For these people, eating any of these foods in even the smallest quantity can cause significant gastric upset. They may have loose stool, bloating, and experience other gastrointestinal upset symptoms. Severe allergy to nightshades can even cause anaphylaxis and even death. This is very rare, and if you had not died after eating a slice of pizza, I think you are in the clear. If, however, you notice that you routinely feel bloated and uncomfortable after eating any of the aforementioned foods, you may want to see if complete elimination of these foods from your diet makes you feel more comfortable. You know your body better than anyone else. If you must eliminate these foods from your diet, do not be concerned because there are several other excellent sources for the nutrients. It would be best if you kept the inflammation in your body to a minimum.

Nothing in medicine is ever clear-cut! Despite the fact that nightshades can cause gastric upset in a small fraction of people, they are so rich in many nutrients that can help fight eye diseases. Nightshades have a high level of antioxidants that we know help protect the eyes against many diseases, from age-related macular degeneration to cataracts. Specifically, tomatoes and bell peppers are very high in beta-carotene, a derivative of vitamin A. This vitamin does a great job of defending our eyes against the many toxins we encounter daily. Furthermore, tomatoes and eggplants are especially high in lutein and zeaxanthin, which we discussed in detail in our macular degeneration section. These highly colorful substances help give the back part of our eye the orange-red color and act as a pair of sunglasses to ensure that the sun's damaging rays do not damage our eyes.

Of the plants in the nightshade family, white potatoes are probably the least healthy. White potatoes are a fruit of our Earth and have a decent amount of potassium, vitamin C, and vitamin B6. However, it would not be my first choice of food in a healthy diet. Because potatoes are digested so quickly, they can cause quick increases in sugar in our blood which contributes to diabetes and obesity. Therefore, if you have your choice between white potatoes and sweet potatoes, I suggest sweet potatoes all day long. This is one of the few instances when something that is sweet for you is actually better than its not-so-sweet counterpart!

What makes nightshades so perplexing is the possibility of inflammation as a result of consuming this food. If you have an inflammatory condition such as rheumatoid arthritis, systemic lupus erythematosus, or multiple sclerosis, or if you think your body does not tolerate nightshades, eliminate them from your body for a month and see how you feel. If you feel better after eliminating this food, then you should not consume nightshades. If you feel no different after elimination for a month, then you are probably not nightshade-sensitive, and you can enjoy the benefits of these highly nutritious foods.

Other Potential Culprits

I am going to prep you here: our discussion around legumes, nuts, and seeds will sound very similar to our talk about bell peppers and tomatoes. The long and short of it here is that several foods can cause inflammation even though they have highly nutritious properties. Nothing in life is ever simple, right!

In case you are unfamiliar with the term legume, I am referring to beans. How about that old song that grandpa used to sing? "Beans, beans, such a wonderful fruit . . ." Well, you know how it ends. There is so much truth that beans provide movement in the digestive system as their fiber content is extremely high. They are also packed with tons of vitamins and minerals. What makes beans tricky is that they are one of the many foods out there that can cause inflammation in some people's digestive tract.

If you think that you are sensitive to beans, nuts, and seeds, try the elimination technique where you simply omit these foods from your diet entirely for a month and reassess your symptoms. If you feel better, then keep those foods out of your diet. If you don't feel better, then go ahead and indulge in all of the nutritious properties these foods offer.

There are many ways that beans, nuts, and seeds can help improve the health of your eyes. The two main areas we will concentrate on are feeding our gut with fibrous prebiotics and reducing inflammation with omega-3 fatty acids.

Fiber is probably the most obvious of the benefits as we all know how well beans help move things along your digestive tract fairly nicely. You may be wondering why fiber is so good for the eyes. You may remember how there is a direct connection between your eyes and your stomach. Your entire nervous system is closely connected to the digestive tract. Scientists call the gut-brain axis, which is a big fancy term for "Your tummy and your brain actually communicate with one another." Your tummy is covered with bacteria that help extract nutrients from food and protect the body. Fiber acts as food for these bacteria to stick around longer and do their job to improve our health. Because fiber helps the bacteria grow, they are called a "prebiotic." When you have a healthy gut, your entire body is healthier, including your eyes.

Omega-3 fatty acids and other nutrients in legumes, nuts, and seeds are important for eye health and brain development. A handful of nuts and seeds is jam-packed with omega-3 fatty acids, which helps to reduce inflammation all over the body. Some nuts are more nutritious than others. But if you can just grab a big handful of nuts a couple of times a day, you will be on your way to a better brain and longer life.

What is White, Grainy, and More Addictive than Cocaine?

SUGAR!

You are probably thinking that I am exaggerating just a bit. Well, I am not. In animal studies, rats were given the choice of water that contained either cocaine or an intense, calorie-free sweetener called saccharin. Believe it or not, the rats chose the sweetener over cocaine 94 percent of the time! Of course, I know rats are not humans. They have not legalized cocaine for a study like this in humans, but I am sure far too many people would probably sign up for the study if they did. In any case, the work of these scientists exemplifies the potentially addictive nature of sugar and added sweeteners.

When we talk about sugar here, we are not talking about the naturally occurring sugar that you find in fruit. The sugar in fruit is an entirely different topic for the next chapter. Right now, we are talking about sugar that is purposely added to foods by food manufacturers supposedly to help preserve food and improve taste. Food manufacturers know that added sugar is highly addictive. So, since they want you to buy more of their product, they add just enough unnatural sugar to get you hooked. And to think that we fall for their trick every time we grab a soda or a bag of chips!

There are so many places where food manufacturers sneak in this added sugar it could make your head spin. Starting with the obvious, most sodas, cookies, and ice cream have added sugar, which is not surprising because all of these treats are sweet. But a food does not need to be sweet to contain added sugar. For instance, most chips, breads, sauces, salad dressings, and processed foods contain some amount of added sugar. Added sugar is literally everywhere and next to impossible to completely avoid.

Since we have added sugar in almost everything we eat and Americans are not dying like hotcakes, what is the big problem? The problem is that people are dying from their sugar intake, and the risk involved with excess sugar in our diet is not ingrained in our heads enough. A study looked at adults in the United States, and they found that over fifteen years, those who got 17–21 percent of their calories from added sugar had a 38 percent increased risk of dying from heart disease! So, you can see that Americans are dying from sugar overconsumption. It is just taking about fifteen years for it to happen.

At this point, we know the close link that diabetes has with eye health. In fact, one out of every four people who have diabetes has a visual impairment—about twice that of those people without diabetes. There have been many studies that have looked at sugar overconsumption in diabetic patients. One study took 310,819 people who researchers deemed as drinking lots of sugary drinks every day. For the purposes of this study, "lots of sugary drinks" was considered anything over two sugary drinks per day. They found that the people who drank two or more sugary drinks per day had a 26 percent greater risk of developing diabetes than those who drank less than two drinks per day. It is amazing to me that two measly sugary drinks can have such a big impact on your health.

If that is not compelling enough, sugar promotes the inflammatory process that we talked about in almost every section thus far. Inflammation kills every system of your body, and sugar puts this process on steroids. So, from your eyes to your heart, we must control the amount of added sugar in our diet to stop inflammation's destruction.

To give us an idea of how much added sugar we should have in our diet, the World Health Organization (WHO) and the 2015–2020 Dietary Guidelines for Americans came up with some very specific parameters to help Americans control sugar intake. These well-accredited teams stated that Americans should make sure that no more than 10 percent of all calories consumed daily are from added sugar. You may have no clue how many calories you consume daily. You are probably saying to yourself, "Now they are asking me to track how many calories I eat from added sugar?" As my Aunt Irma, who is straight out of Queens, would say, "Fuhgeddaboudit!" If you follow the *Beyond Carrots* Plan, you will definitely be in the less than 10 percent range for added sugar. If you are not completely ready to dive headfirst into the *Beyond Carrots* Plan, I get it. Let's just start by cutting back your sugary drinks to less than two per day. This will put you on track for a healthier life and reduced risk of blindness.

An Apple a Day Keeps the Doctor Away

Would you believe that there is actually some truth to this adage? The main reason we are talking about fruit is to introduce them as a healthy alternative to refined sugar. Sometimes that sugar craving will drive us insane, but by turning to fruit, we can get that same sort of satisfaction without the toxic side effects. In fact, by replacing one cookie or cola per day with an apple, one could make a significant difference in their blood sugar levels. That is not to mention the number of vitamins, minerals, and fiber in a single piece of fruit.

Immunity Booster

As it relates to the eyes, one of the key benefits of including fruit in your diet is to boost your natural vitamin C intake. When we think about this vitamin, the first thing we think of is usually its cold-fighting powers. Vitamin C does a ton of amazing things in the eyes, from helping to delay the onset of cataracts to protecting the eyes against macular degeneration. Vitamin C is considered an antioxidant, and we have talked extensively about the importance of antioxidants in reversing eye disease. Fruits like pineapple, mango, lemons, and, of course, oranges are jam-packed with vitamin C. We don't hear as much about guava, but it is another fantastic source of vitamin C.

Cancer-Fighting

There are a ton of other antioxidants present in fruit that help boost immunity and defend our bodies against infection. Lycopene, lutein, and beta-carotene are just a few examples of the antioxidants present in fruit. Lycopene has been in the spotlight recently for its superb cancer-fighting superpowers. You can find this rockstar highly concentrated in papaya, apple, and watermelon.

Blood Lipid Level/Blood Pressure Control

What if I told you that you could reduce fat in your body and help control your blood pressure by eating fruit? Believe it or not, lemons can help lower your blood lipid levels and control your blood pressure. Lemon water has also been shown to be incredibly powerful in reducing kidney stones. How amazing is it that you can help control your weight by simply adding a little lemon to your water throughout the day!

Control Insulin Resistance/Cholesterol Level

Grapefruit has been shown to aid in insulin resistance which can help those patients with diabetes. Grapefruit can also help to reduce cholesterol levels. Anything that you can do to help control blood sugar and cholesterol levels will positively impact your eye health. I would like to mention a word of caution around grapefruit. There are some medications that do not mesh well with grapefruit, so make sure you talk to your primary care doctor before you load up on this citrus fruit.

Potassium

Including adequate potassium intake in your diet can have a significant impact on your heart and eye health. Specifically, potassium helps to reduce your risk of cardiovascular disease and stroke. Did you know that you can get a stroke in your eye? I have seen it happen, and it is not a pretty thing. Perhaps something slightly more relatable is the infamous eye twitch. Have you ever had a bout of eye twitches that just won't go away? Potassium has been said to help control this twitching. I would also add a little meditation or stress-relieving activities as the twitching, often, has a stress component. Fruit is an excellent source of potassium. Two fruits that are most easily attainable that have incredible amounts of potassium are bananas and apples.

Prebiotic

Remember our long conversation around gut health? Well, eating fruit is like feeding the good bacteria in our tummies so that they can flourish. In the medical world, we call the foods that feed our good bacteria prebiotics. What happens is that the prebiotics turn into a jelly-like substance when it gets to the gut, and the good bacteria start smiling ear to ear because it is feast time.

The specific prebiotic that is present in many fruits is pectin. Pectin is called a soluble fiber because when it sucks in water, it turns super sticky, and the gut is in heaven. This soluble fiber helps keep our gut healthy and our immune system strong. Many fruits have a high pectin concentration, but apples are one of the most popular. I bet you are starting to realize why an apple a day keeps the doctor away.

An Apple a Day ...

It takes a lot for a single serving of fruit to get the reputation of keeping the doctor away. Apples truly are a mega fruit with so many benefits that we have already discussed packed into each bite. They are packed with fiber and prebiotics that feed those good bacteria in our gut. Apples have a high potassium content to help protect our hearts, reduce the risk of strokes, and minimize those annoying eye twitches. They also have super high vitamin C content and antioxidants galore. If that's not enough, apples help to reduce the risk of type 2 diabetes. A review of forty-one studies went so far as to say that those people who ate more apples actually had a reduced risk of developing lung cancer. That is a pretty powerful fruit!

How about an All-Fruit Diet?

With all the health benefits that fruit provides, it sounds like you should just be able to eat an all-fruit diet and cure every ailment. Not so fast; there is something else we must talk about—good old glycemic index. The glycemic index is a measure of how fast foods impact your body's blood sugar level. Lower glycemic index fruits such as cherries and grapefruit impact your body's blood sugar level very slowly. High glycemic index fruits such as bananas and pineapples cause a sharp increase in your body's blood sugar level. As a general rule of thumb, the sweeter the fruit, the higher the glycemic index.

The technical term for having too much sugar in the body is "hyperglycemia." Being in this state of high blood sugar for any length of time can cause damage to every organ of your body. Anyone who has diabetes has heard about this damage since the first time they heard the word "diabetes."

The eyes are a prime target for damage due to hyperglycemia. Having high blood sugar can cause blurred vision and changes in your glasses prescription. If the blood sugar level gets high enough, you can damage the nerves in the back part of the eye. You also have double the risk of developing glaucoma when your blood sugar is out of control as it is a diabetic patient.

The bottom line here is that although fruit has some amazing benefits on your body and eyes, it cannot be a standalone food for a rich and balanced diet. It is best to be aware of how much fruit you include in your diet and the sweetness of those fruits. You can go so far as to look up their glycemic index, but this may be overkill. If you follow the guidelines in the *Beyond Carrots* Plan, you will be on your way to a healthier body and eyes without an overload of apples and bananas each day.

What do British Fighter Pilots and Carrots Have in Common?

One of the questions that I get most often as an optometrist specializing in anti-aging medicine and nutrition is, "Are carrots really good for your eyes?" The quick and simple answer to this question is YES!

As you recall, carrots became popularized as the vegetable that miraculously improved eyesight during World War II. During the war, the British developed special technology that helped them see at night. The fighter pilots wanted to keep their technology a secret but knew that people might notice that their pilots could see better at night, so they created propaganda around the idea that their pilots were eating carrots to help improve their eyesight. As an added benefit to starting this rumor, the Brits hoped that they might encourage the massive number of people who were living in poverty during the war to eat carrots—a cheap, nutritious food. Their propaganda worked, and carrots are still known as an eye superfood today.

Ironically enough, there is some truth to the idea that carrots are good for the eyes. If you recall our discussion about the back part of the eye and the macula, you may remember that this structure is an orange-red color. What makes it this hue is the pigment that is so highly concentrated in this area. Foods like carrots and spinach are high in vitamin A, lutein, and other phytonutrients that help serve to defend our eyes against diseases like macular degeneration. Pretty much any vegetable that has color to it will help protect the eyes due to its high level of antioxidants, including vitamin A.

The bottom line around carrots is that they are great for the eyes, but I would not recommend them as a sole source of eye nutrition. Variety is the spice of life, so add some flair to your diet.

Popeye was a Smart Man

Popeye certainly knew what he was doing when he routinely popped open that can of spinach. I am pretty sure that if he were not in a pinch for time, Popeye would have chosen to eat fresh or sautéed spinach, but canned is better than nothing! Let's talk about why spinach is considered an eye superfood.

If you were to look back on the last chapter when we talked about the antioxidant levels of various foods, you would see that spinach is very high on this list. If you did not have this list in front of you when you were at the grocery store trying to decide what vegetable to eat for dinner, you should pick out which foods are highest in antioxidants based on the color of the vegetable. In general, the foods that are darkest green or brightest in colors are usually the foods that are highest in phytonutrients that help protect the eyes. In the vegetable aisle, you may notice that kale and spinach are darker green than romaine and iceberg lettuce. Ding, ding, ding! You got it; kale and spinach are far superior for your eyes than romaine and iceberg.

As a side note, spinach is not necessarily a muscle-building food as it is depicted with our friendly sailor. Even though green leafy vegetables should be included in our diet every day in an attempt to protect the eyes, we are much better off turning to protein to build muscle. Nevertheless, Popeye was still on the right track and a smart man for his excellent choice in foods!

The Anti-Cancer Food

An integral part of the *Beyond Carrots* Plan is a group of vegetables called the cruciferous vegetables. This group of vegetables has been in the spotlight recently for its possible anti-cancer properties. While anti-cancer may be a little bit of a stretch, we will discuss the health benefits of these superfoods and why they are so important in your *Beyond Carrots* Plan.

Here are some examples of cruciferous vegetables, so you know what we are talking about here:

- Brussel sprouts
- Broccoli
- Bok choy
- Cabbage
- Cauliflower
- Collard greens
- Kale
- Radish
- Horseradish

As you go through that list of vegetables, there is one thing that they have in common. They all have that characteristically pungent smell and bitter taste that can be attributed to the fact that they have a sulfur-containing compound, and sulfur stinks! You know what I am talking about!

It is also interesting to note that cruciferous vegetables got their name from the Latin word for cross, *crucifix*. Supposedly, the reason why the vegetable naming people landed on this name is because the flowers of this plant are in the shape of a cross. Personally, I do not see where they look like a cross, but I guess that does not matter.

So, let's dive into the many reasons why this foul-smelling yet yummy group of vegetables has made it to the list of foods that we must eat on the *Beyond Carrots* Plan.

Possible Cancer-Fighting Properties

We talk about the cancer-fighting powers in cruciferous vegetables very loosely. I do not want to build up your hopes that you are going to be able to reverse your lung cancer by eating broccoli. That just isn't happening. However, some important points must be addressed when we talk about the benefits of these vegetables.

Cruciferous vegetables have been in the spotlight recently because a number of studies in rats demonstrate the ability of these vegetables to protect the rats against cancer. The researchers attribute this finding to a component of cruciferous vegetables called glucosinolates. It is the glucosinolates that break down to sulfa. In addition to stinking up the room, the byproducts of glucosinolates are said to be cancer-protective in nature.

Now, the results of these studies are still being researched in humans. One particularly compelling study is the Nurses' Health Study and Health Professional Follow-up Study. Here we find that women who ate more than five servings of cruciferous vegetables per week had lower lung cancer. That is pretty amazing! Although we cannot take the anti-cancer properties as gospel, it is important to note these possible benefits as we consider why we are eating so much broccoli and cauliflower on the *Beyond Carrots* Plan.

Cardiovascular Health

The benefits of cruciferous vegetables on cardiovascular health are very much well-substantiated. Countless studies show that if you eat your broccoli and brussels sprouts, you will have better heart health. One of the largest studies on this topic was based out of my favorite city in China, Shanghai. The Shanghai Women's Health Study and Shanghai Men's Health Study took 134,796 people and looked at how eating cruciferous vegetables affected death. They found that those who ate the most cruciferous vegetables had a 22 percent reduced risk of dying in general and 31 percent reduced risk of dying from cardiovascular disease, compared to those people who hardly ate any of these vegetables at all. In case you are not sure what I mean by cardiovascular disease, I am talking about anything that affects the heart and blood flow from heart attack to stroke.

There have been a number of similar studies that we do not need to dive into because you do not want to hear about studies all day. The bottom line is that scientists have some pretty convincing research on how cruciferous vegetables benefit heart health. So, although this is an eye book, we are going to include broccoli and cauliflower in our plan. Your eyes are useless if you are dead because your heart is not healthy.

Gut Health

Remember that what happens in the gut affects our entire body. When you have a happy gut, you have a happy body. Cruciferous vegetables are like fertile soil for the good bacteria in the gut. When we eat these vegetables, the good bacteria in the gut multiply and thrive. The high fiber content of vegetables like cauliflower and broccoli plays a key role in keeping our tummies happy. These fiber-rich foods form a gooey, gelatinous substance. When it hits the gut like a big cozy, fluffy blanket, our gut feels like it died and went to heaven.

Brain Function

What if I took the amazing benefits of cruciferous vegetables one step further and told you that you could actually slow the aging process in your brain by eating increasing your consumption of these nutrient-rich veggies? Researchers at Brigham and Woman's Hospital in Boston, Massachusetts, did just that. They took 13,388 women from their hospital and found that those people who ate the most cruciferous vegetables had the slowest decline in cognitive function. This does not surprise me in the least. These vegetables are super high in their lutein and zeaxanthin content. Lutein and zeaxanthin are some of the few nutrients that can pass right on into the brain and protect the brain against damage.

Eye Health

Last but not least, cruciferous vegetable consumption is the cornerstone for maintaining excellent eye health. These vegetables are incredibly high in carotenoids such as beta-carotene, lutein, and zeaxanthin. These are the key nutrients that help to detoxify the eye. They go so far as to reverse damage to the back part of the eye and reduce the risk of developing macular degeneration. The efforts of key carotenoids are backed by the high vitamin C content in these veggies. Vitamin C is like a super antioxidant and is critical for stellar eye health.

The Pee-You Power

From the times of ancient civilization, the power of garlic has been used to heal. The Romans, Greeks, Chinese, and even the Egyptians recognized garlic for its ability to help fight disease. Garlic has a distinct smell that we all know and love, especially if you are eating at my Aunt Irma's house. The compound in garlic that gives it this pungent odor is sulfur. Ironically enough, this same compound gives garlic its wide array of health benefits that we are going to utilize in our *Beyond Carrots* Plan.

First of all, garlic is a natural antibiotic and antiviral. When either applied topically or ingested, garlic will kill bad bacteria and viruses that it comes across. I cannot imagine that it would be comfortable to put garlic in the eye. I would strongly discourage you from trying to do this at home. However, a study conducted in Africa revealed that garlic was as effective as some antibiotic drops at curing eye infections. We are not going to be putting garlic in the eye; rather, we will be using garlic's antibiotic properties to maintain a healthy body and digestive tract.

Garlic's powerful boost to our bodies' immune system is like pulling out the very best defense troops we can find. There may be no cure for the common cold but eating the right foods will certainly get your body better equipped to fight off infections. The efficacy of garlic in protecting the body was investigated in a twelve-week study where they found that daily garlic consumption in the form of a pill reduced the number of colds by 63 percent compared to a group who took the placebo. So now you are starting to understand why garlic is so important in your *Beyond Carrots* Plan.

Furthermore, garlic is packed with powerful antioxidants. We know, by now, that consuming antioxidants protects the body, brain, and eyes. This helps to delay the aging process in every square inch of our bodies. You could go so far as to say that garlic is an anti-aging superfood.

Garlic also can lower cholesterol, modulate blood sugar, and reduce blood pressure. In addition, it has been demonstrated that garlic is as effective as atenolol, a popular blood pressure-lowering drug, at reducing blood pressure. Now, I am not telling you to eat garlic and stop all meds. What I am saying is that by consuming garlic on a daily basis, we are going to be well on our way to a healthier version of you!

Battle of Land and Sea

Vegetarian, paleo, vegan, pescatarian . . . the fad diet alphabet soup could go on and on. We could get so caught up in the different options out there in a search to have the healthiest diet possible. I will go ahead and spill the beans for you before we even start talking about the battle of land and sea. The best diet for you is the diet that fits YOUR lifestyle and fitness goals. At the end of the day, you have to feel good about yourself and what you ate that day. It's as simple as that! But, as my dad always says, "Knowledge is power," so let's try to break these diet restrictions down for you.

If you were to do absolutely nothing and eat like most Americans eat, you would be eating a SAD (Standard American Diet). Americans are not necessarily well-known for their diet plan. If you close your eyes and picture an American cookout, you may find hot dogs, chips, soft drinks, potato salad, and cake. Everything on this menu is either processed or full of sugar. If you were forced to pick a diet for the rest of your life, I recommend you research other options.

Let's take a trip to Italy for a minute. Who doesn't love the luscious countryside of Italy? In case you did not gather this from my name, I am Italian. My dad came to America on a boat from Italy when he was nine years old. We still have strong family connections in Italy, and we go back to see our relatives overseas annually. As a quick refresher on geography, this region is near the Mediterranean Sea, so the food they eat is called the Mediterranean Diet.

When my dad grew up in the countryside, sugar was very expensive, but olives were plentiful. They had lots of tomatoes, beans, and vegetables, but meat was scarce. For a special holiday, they may find a rabbit, and that one rabbit would feed a family of eight. I am sure this sounds quite different than our diets in America. Dad did not come to America for the food, I assure you of that!

The vegetarian diet consists solely of vegetables. The skeptic may wonder how one can get all of the protein needed in your diet from vegetables alone. But believe it or not, it's possible!

If you were to ask five different doctors about the best eating pattern for a healthy life, you would probably get five different opinions. I will tell you what I did when I was trying to reverse my eye disease. I am not saying that this is the only way to live a healthy life and feel great, but it worked for me.

My eye disease-crushing eating plan consisted of foods that grow in or on the land or sea. What I mean by that is that I ate only fruit, vegetables, meat, and seafood. I eliminated all dairy, eggs, bread, and pasta. I also eliminated anything that was white such as white potatoes and white rice. These foods are not nutrient-dense and can contribute to inflammation. Instead, I loaded up on healthy starches such as sweet potato, quinoa, and brown rice.

When I was trying to reverse my eye disease, I was under a stringent time crunch given the potentially progressive nature of my condition. I had to be diligent about my strict diet, and I could not cheat even once. Sunday dinner with my Italian family was very awkward when I told my Aunt Irma that I could not eat pasta. I was lucky enough to be able to get everything under control in thirty days. Some people may take ninety to one hundred and twenty days to get their inflammatory condition under control. It is important to stick with it and not cheat even once until you are positive your condition has reversed. Cheating once can throw you off, and you will end up back on square one.

After you have gotten to the point where your disease is under control, an occasional pasta dinner is not going to kill you. Ideally, you would stick with the strict diet sixty days before having your first cheat day. You will be amazed at how good you feel! It would not surprise me if you lose a little weight eating like this. It is hard to put on serious pounds eating chicken, brown rice, and broccoli.

America Really Does Run on Coffee!

If not for our morning joe, Americans would be dumber, heavier, and die at a younger age. Now *that* is a reason to drink your coffee! The list of health benefits linked to coffee consumption is lengthy, but we will talk about some of the most important benefits of this amazing drink.

To start, your morning joe gives you that caffeine boost that many of us crave. This, in turn, boosts our mood as research has shown that coffee can make you happier. In addition, coffee improves brain function and memory. One amazing study showed that coffee drinkers had a 65 percent reduced risk of developing Alzheimer's. (Maybe my mom should start drinking more coffee so she stops repeating herself so much.)

Coffee can help modulate blood sugar, too. Researchers determined that those people who drink coffee have a 23–50 percent lower risk of developing diabetes. One study took 457,922 people and looked at the effects of coffee on their risk of developing diabetes. They found that each cup of coffee reduced the risk of developing diabetes by 7 percent. That is some powerful stuff. As we know, one of the first places that diabetes attacks is the back part of the eyes.

Pretty much everyone I know loves to burn fat. Did you know that coffee is a natural fat burner? You can say goodbye to those overpriced supplements with this inexpensive power horse. The scientists studied this only to find that coffee increases fat burning in those people that are obese by 10 percent and those who are lean by 29 percent. I know you are going to ask me why the disparity between the obese and lean. Quite frankly, I have no good answer.

If you have ever had a cup of coffee before you hit the gym, you probably notice that you can push yourself just a little bit harder. You may take one more crunch or add that extra ten pounds to your set, just for kicks and giggles. Coffee gives you a slight adrenaline rush through a substance called epinephrine which initiates the "fight or flight" response, which results in heightened physical performance. So, drink a cup of joe before you hit the gym and see for yourself.

The phytochemicals in coffee are even anti-aging. Coffee is jam-packed with nutrients that help to slow down the aging process and protect the eyes. The name for these antioxidants in coffee is polyphenols. Coffee has been recognized as number eleven in the list of one hundred richest dietary sources of polyphenols. Some studies go so far as to say that Americans get more antioxidants from coffee than fruits and vegetables combined.

Not all coffee is created equal. As soon as you load your drink with cream, sugar, and other artificial sweeteners, you negate the beneficial effects of this powerful drink. I totally understand that black coffee is an acquired taste. I started drinking my coffee black because I was so busy at work, I did not have time to add milk and sugar. For those of you who cannot drink black coffee, I have a couple of suggestions. First, head for milk that is just a little less fatty than whatever you are used to. If you are currently drinking cream, try whole milk. If you are currently drinking whole milk, try two percent. The goal here is to ween your way away from the fat. Second, instead of tons of and other artificial sweeteners, turn to natural sweeteners such as monk fruit.

I am not advising that you drink ten cups of coffee a day. Too much of anything is not a good thing. Furthermore, certain people need to be careful about their coffee consumption. For instance, coffee can elevate your blood pressure, especially if you already have high blood pressure. So, if you are taking blood pressure medications or have been told you are hypertensive, talk to your doctor about the amount of coffee you drink. Likewise, if you have GERD (gastroesophageal reflux disease), Crohn's disease, frequent heartburn, or digestive issues, you should talk to your doctor about drinking coffee before you overindulge. Coffee can exacerbate these conditions and cause much discomfort. On a similar note, if you already have trouble sleeping, you may want to cut back on coffee to see if your sleeping improves because caffeine can have a serious impact on your sleep patterns. Make sure you drink your coffee early in the day and switch to water in the afternoon.

You may wonder why some "cleanses" omit coffee. Coffee can impact the cleansing of the liver when trying to do a complete flush of all toxins. The *Beyond Carrots* Plan is not a cleanse; it is a complete lifestyle change. This is not something that you do one week and then move on. For some people, omitting coffee from their lives would be next to impossible. Who would want to do that anyway with all the health benefits of this powerful drink?

In the *Beyond Carrots* Plan, I recommend that you try to keep coffee consumption to around one or two cups of coffee daily. Some coffee is good for you, but if you are pounding coffee all day long, you may want to cut back. Our goal here is to improve your mental state, reduce blood sugar, improve your workout, slow down the aging process, and, of course, protect the eyes.

Jewish Penicillin

When you are sick with a runny nose, sore throat, and fever, what is the first food that comes to your mind? Chicken soup! What is it about the chicken soup that is so amazing for you? Is it the chicken in the soup? Is it the celery and carrots? Could it be the diced-up onions? Although each of the ingredients in chicken soup adds to its ability to help soothe illnesses, research has shown that chicken broth is a powerful tool in our disease-fighting arsenal. There is a reason why Jewish people call chicken soup "Jewish Penicillin."

The broth in chicken soup is typically the bone broth made from chicken bones. It is important to note that the healing broth we are talking about here is bone broth, not vegetable broth. Broth made from chicken or beef bones contains easily-absorbed nutrients that can help repair our bodies from the inside out.

Making bone broth is super easy! All you need to do is throw about three pounds of bones with about eight to ten cups of water and a bit of apple cider vinegar in your Crock-Pot for eight to ten hours. You can always throw in some carrots, celery, onion, salt, and pepper for flavor. If you don't have a Crock-Pot, you can always cook it on the stove. The main point is that you need to cook on low for a very long time. After eight to ten hours, strain with a fine-mesh strainer, and you will end up with around five cups of pure goodness. You can either freeze for about three months or refrigerate and drink within a couple of days. If you were wondering, you can usually pick up bones at your local butcher shop or your grocery store in the meat section. I, personally, love to use the carcass from a roasted chicken because it's quick, easy, and flavorful.

Bone broth is especially healing because it is jam-packed with our bodies' building blocks. These building blocks are called amino acids, and their presence can affect so much, from our ability to fight off infection to obtaining a restful night of sleep. The two amino acids that we are going to focus on here are glutamine and glycine. The slow cooking process of making broth allows these key players to be released into the liquid and become extremely easy for our bodies to absorb. Let's dive into the nitty-gritty about what these healing elements can do for our bodies.

Bone broth is packed with glutamine, a powerful player in the anti-inflammatory world because it helps calm the inflammatory storm throughout the body. From our gut to our brain, glutamine makes it happen. The biggest challenge with this amino acid is getting it absorbed into the body. If you were to try to take glutamine in pill form, most of it would probably end up in the toilet because it passes right through the body. The glutamine in bone broth passes right into your body and is super effective at reducing inflammation.

Another key player in bone broth, glycine, has been shown to improve sleep patterns. Research shows that the glycine found in bone broth can help you fall asleep faster, stay asleep longer, and achieve a deeper sleep throughout the evening. To get the biggest bang for your buck from this sleep aid, pass on the evening glass of wine and pour a delicious cup of bone broth. You will be amazed at how fabulous you feel in the morning!

If that is not enough, bone broth helps aid in weight loss. Bone broth fills you up quickly because it is a liquid that is high in protein and relatively low in calories. This gives you the feeling of being full without eating a ton because your little tummy is full of fluid. Unlike juice cleanses that fill you up with liquid with little to no protein, bone broth will not deprive your body of its essential building blocks.

The beneficial effects of bone broth will ultimately improve your eyes along with your body. Therefore, bone broth is a vital part of the *Beyond Carrots* Plan. You will begin to feel the effects of this healing agent within two weeks of starting the program. You will be amazed at how the warm, soothing nature of the broth eases tension and promotes relaxation.

What Color is Your Urine?

What color is your urine? A super quick and easy way to determine how dehydrated you are is by looking at the color of your urine. If you notice that your urine is a deep yellow color, you are probably not drinking enough water. If your urine is practically clear, you are well hydrated. Our goal is always to consume enough water to keep our urine clear to prevent dehydration.

It may surprise you that dehydration can have a big impact on your eye health. This is because a dry body leads to dry eyes. As a result, you may experience all of the signs and symptoms of dry eye, including redness, burning, tearing, headaches, and pain around the eyes. Often, the easiest way to fix dryness is by increasing the amount of water you drink daily.

Water also assists in cleaning the body of its waste; it helps get rid of toxins. In other words, water helps you poop. If you are constipated or do not poop too often, you probably don't ingest enough of Mother Earth's finest resource. Constipation and the buildup of toxins in the body can exacerbate autoimmune disorders such as multiple sclerosis and rheumatoid arthritis. You may recall from our talks about autoimmune disorders: if they are present in one location, they are all over the body. Autoimmune disorders are like cockroaches. You never find them in just one place, and your eye is a prime spot for these disorders to attack.

There are all sorts of formulas out there that calculate how much water should be consumed daily to remain adequately hydrated. Some people say that you should drink half of your body weight in ounces daily. Others give exact formulas for determining how much water should be consumed. However, there is no exact science as to how much you should drink. It depends on your physical activity, heat exposure, and diet. For instance, if you were in the sun all day doing manual labor and had a salty cheese pizza for dinner, you are definitely going to be dehydrated and should increase your water intake. Using the formulas as a guideline is great but be sure to adjust based on your individual needs. I still maintain that the best way to assess your water intake level is by grading your urine color.

By the way, there are so many ways to add flair to boring water. Infusing fruit into water has become popular over the past few years. You can even find special devices that aid in the infusion of fruits, vegetables, and herbs into your water. It can be so much fun to experiment with a flavor combination. You don't even need one of those fancy infusers to explore the fun world of flavored water. Just get a pitcher and add a combo of fruits, vegetables, and herbs. Then just let it soak for a couple of hours. You will be amazed at how fast you down that water when it tastes delicious and is packed with nutrients.

How to Drink Like an Italian

If you have never been to Italy, let me tell you about how they drink their alcohol. There is no such thing as a family meal in Italy without a glass of wine. This means that Italians drink wine pretty much daily. In America, a person who drinks every day may be classified as an alcoholic. What differentiates the Italians' drinking from the Americans' drinking is the size of the glass and the number of glasses that they drink. The glass of wine that accompanies the pasta dinner in Italy is just a little bigger than a shot glass. In other words, it is very tiny, and you would need about three Italian glasses to fill one American glass of wine. There is a lot of goodness packed into those precious sips of *"vino,"* from protecting the heart to reducing inflammation. The challenge here is to remember that American culture has normalized overdrinking, and in order to reap the health benefits of wine, we must drink like the Italians.

CDC reports indicate that 17 percent of American adults admitted to binge drinking a minimum of once per week in 2015. That means that the average American had approximately fifty-three binge drinking nights over the course of the year, with binge drinking categorized as anything over seven drinks per night.

"The French Paradox" is one of my favorite terms to describe the power of wine. Despite the high level of saturated fat intake among the overall French population, the level of heart attacks, otherwise known as ischemic heart disease, is incredibly low. Researchers attribute the low level of death from the high-fat diet to the consumption of red wine. My mom would be thrilled if she heard about this finding, and she would just drink some red wine with her fried chicken, and she would be loving life.

But it is not that simple. Wine certainly has some fantastic benefits and is most well-known for its cardioprotective abilities, commonly attributed to one of its key players, resveratrol. Resveratrol and proanthocyanins are powerful antioxidants found in wine that help to prevent cardiovascular problems like stroke and heart attacks.

Resveratrol researchers took things one step further and looked closely at its ability to reduce inflammation. They analyzed a group of 2,900 women who drank moderately and found that they had lower inflammatory risk factors over a period of eight years. This research supports the idea that resveratrol in red wine protects our hearts and reduces blood clots. I will drink to that!

Here's another one of my favorite wine studies. A group of scientists took 5,505 people and found that those who had two to seven drinks per week had lower rates of depression. What is key to note in this study is that they are not talking about two to seven drinks per *night*. That will not make you happy!

With All Those Positive Effects, What Could Go Wrong with Alcohol and the Eyes?

Many things could go wrong when you drink alcohol, especially as it relates to eye health. I know that many people would love to hear that alcohol is a great thing to add to your daily diet. As you can see from the studies listed above, there are some beneficial effects when drank in very small quantities. However, there is a thin line between a small drink and overindulging. The list of complications from overindulging in alcohol is pretty extensive, so brace yourself. You may want to grab your last drink before you read this section. You are not going to want a drink when you are done.

Central Nervous System Damage

Perhaps one of the most notable problems with alcohol is the damage to the central nervous system that occurs when you drink. As you probably realize by now, the eyes are connected to the central nervous system. I hope that you have never been pulled over for a DUI, but if you have, you may have noticed that the police officer shines a light in your eyes and looks at eye movement. They are looking at eye movement because when you drink too much, your eyes start to wiggle as they move. This wiggling is a reflection of your loss of motor control and is called nystagmus. If you lose control of eye movement with alcohol consumption, it is no wonder why driving under the influence can be dangerous.

To make matters worse, the eyes are supposed to constrict when exposed to light and dilate or become larger when in the dark. A fancier name for this phenomenon is called a pupillary light response. The pupils' ability to respond to light is dependent on a functioning central nervous system. Damage to this part of the brain with drinking causes your pupils not to constrict properly. So, when you are driving in the dark at night and see an oncoming headlight under the influence of alcohol, your eyes do not respond properly, and you cannot see worth a darn. Boom! Car crash. *No bueno.*

Permanent Death of the Optic Nerve

In light of the previous problems with driving and alcohol consumption, let's just say that you decide to stay home and drink. What could go wrong, right? Wrong. Excessive drinking can cause permanent and irreversible death of the nerve that connects the eye to the brain. The technical term for this problem is alcohol amblyopia or tobacco-alcohol amblyopia. The root cause of this vision loss is the nutritional deficiency of vitamin B12, thiamine, folate, and riboflavin related to prolonged heavy alcohol consumption.

Now, you would have to drink a TON for a long period of time in order to get to the point that you have a loss of communication between your brain and your eyes. In fact, studies have shown that as long as you have not been in a vitamin-deficient state for too long, you can simply replace the deficient vitamins, and your vision will return to normal. So, if you wanted to be super sneaky, you could just make sure you supplement with a ton of B vitamins and pray that you are in the clear. However, I would strongly advise against doing this as the effects of alcohol go beyond the death of the optic nerve.

Early Onset Cataract Formation

Prolonged vitamin deficiency related to heavy alcohol consumption goes beyond the brain damage previously discussed. This damage can extend to impact every square inch of your body. Even the tiny lens in your eye that helps to focus light can be affected by vitamin deficiency. When the lens of the eye does not have the proper nutrition, it gets damaged more easily and will experience early onset cataract formation. These cataracts cause extensive glare, halos, and blur.

Full disclosure, I am not dreading my cataract surgery as I know that cataract surgery can correct vision to the point where glasses may not be necessary after the procedure. However, I certainly don't want to do a procedure at an early age and unnecessarily because I drank too much booze. That would be a very expensive drink!

Puffy, Red, Tired-Looking Eyes

If I did not get you on vision loss, perhaps you are vain enough to halt drinking on account of what alcohol does to you aesthetically. If you have ever looked into a person's eyes after a night of heavy drinking, they just look glazed and confused. Alcohol does not make us look prettier. In fact, it ages your body and your eyes.

To begin with, you may notice that the eyelids of heavy drinkers have a sort of puffy appearance. Part of the reason why this happens is that when you overdrink for a long period, your eyelid will enter this state called myokymia, where it has tiny twitches, and this causes puffy eyelids. People in the beauty world spend hours trying to make eyelids less puffy with cucumbers and teabags. This is all destroyed when we overindulge.

Have you ever grabbed your favorite "get the red out" drops after a big night of partying so that your eyes look somewhat normal? Well, these drops can dry the heck out of our eyes, making them appear red, watery, and glossed over. The drops may temporarily help them look less red, but they won't fix the glossed-over appearance that makes you look like you got run over by a car.

You can say, "Shut up, liver! You are fine," after your sixth cocktail and continuous battering of this precious organ of your body. However, if you continue to abuse this vital body part long enough, sooner or later, it will cash out, and you will enter a state of liver damage. Your liver has some very important roles, and when it decides to retire, you can be faced with some very big problems.

For one, your liver is responsible for processing the breakdown products of hemoglobin, our bodies' transporter of oxygen. This product that we are talking about is called bilirubin. When the liver does not clear it, you get a buildup all over the body, and you enter a state called jaundice. This is not a very pretty appearance. Your skin and eyes take on a yellowish tint, and your look unhealthy and pasty. So, give your liver a break on the booze, or you will not be entering a fashion show anytime soon.

Digestive System Damage

I am not telling you anything you do not already know when I tell you alcohol upsets your stomach. If you drink too much, you irritate your digestive system, and you may throw up. It's as simple as that. However, a bigger problem than cleaning up puke is the damage that alcohol does to the digestive system and the malabsorption of nutrients that occurs with drinking.

When you consume excess amounts of alcohol, your stomach lining gets irritated due to the consumption of potentially toxic chemicals in your drink. When your stomach lining gets irritated, the barrier between your gut and the outside world is broken, leaving you exposed to all sorts of infections and an elevated risk of autoimmune disease that can directly impact the eyes. The main point here is that alcohol can make it more difficult for our bodies to fight off infection and may cause the body to start attacking itself via an autoimmune disease. I can tell you firsthand that autoimmune diseases can impact eye health.

If that is not enough, this irritation of the stomach lining also impacts the absorption of nutrients. Your body can't absorb the good things from food when you are consuming and throwing up toxic chemicals.

I think it is clear here that if you can keep your alcohol consumption to a small glass here and there, you will be giving your body a special treat that can help lead to better vision and a longer, happier life. However, if you consume more than a glass or two, you run the risk of doing more harm than good, and your entire body will feel the effects of your careless behavior. My personal recommendation for most Americans is to cut whatever you are drinking in half. That is a solid goal. If you don't drink alcohol, don't start now. All of the benefits of alcohol can be attained with a healthy diet and lifestyle.

Chapter 5:
Lifestyle and Its Impact on Eye Health

A 60 Hour Work Week Can Actually Cause Vision Loss. Tell That to Your Boss!

Believe it or not, excess stress at work and in life can damage your eyes. I would go so far as to say that I faced the possibility of blindness is because I was under a lot of stress at work. For a period of time, I saw patients seven days a week with two days off a month. I am going to tell you something: this is not a healthy lifestyle. When I was told that I could lose my sight and the disease process was autoimmune, I began to connect the dots. I was aware that stress could bring on all sorts of problems, but I never thought that would happen to me. As part of the regimen that I put together to help repair my eyes, I included stress reduction techniques. I will share these techniques with you in section three of this book in hopes that you will incorporate some habits that work for you into your *Beyond Carrots* Plan.

Stress can have a detrimental effect on your eyes in so many ways. I already alluded to the fact that excess pressure in your life can exacerbate autoimmune diseases and inflammation. When your body is in a stress mode, it is gearing up to fight and fend off whatever it finds a threat and releases a hormone called cortisol. A little bit of stress can be good for productivity and mental strength and is called eustress. If this goes on for a long time, your body starts to fight itself in addition to whatever it finds stress in its environment. This is called distress and is at the core of the disease process in autoimmune diseases. Although the list of autoimmune diseases that can affect the eye is extensive, some of the most common are rheumatoid arthritis, systemic lupus erythematous, and dry eye syndrome.

Perhaps the most obvious symptom that your eyes may experience if you are stressed is a twitch of the lid. Almost every time a patient comes into my office with a bouncing eyelid, they have an extreme amount of pressure in their lives. I tell these patients to find some way to decompress daily. They usually look at me as if I have two heads when I try to explain that the importance of meditation and its impact on the body. But, I promise, ten minutes of mindfulness and meditation can really go a long way. I also tell them to eat a banana daily until the spasm stops as bananas are high in potassium, which helps relax the muscles around the eye.

Another eye problem that is linked to stress is called central serous retinopathy. In this condition, a pocket of fluid forms right at the best central vision part of the back part of the eye. Although the annoying bubble back there does not cause blindness, it can reduce the vision to a level where it can become extremely difficult to see. The classic victim of central serous retinopathy is a 30–45-year-old male who is extremely overworked. Again, it sounds so simple, but a lifestyle change is imperative to help reverse this condition.

Since it is clear that too much work and too little relaxation is not good for the eyes, in the *Beyond Carrots* Plan, you will be asked to take a moment to assess the areas of your life where you can minimize tension. You will also be encouraged to find time in your day for activities that reduce cortisol, your body's stress hormone. Speaking from experience, when I changed my work schedule from only having two days off a month to working five days a week, my entire outlook on life changed. I began to enjoy my days at work, and I looked forward to seeing my patients. I also added a simple habit of meditating ten minutes every morning after my workout. I cannot tell you how much I look forward to my mindfulness time. The main takeaway here is that stress impacts every square inch of your body, so you must find ways to manage your life, or you could face vision loss.

If You Can Walk Your Dog, You Can Meditate

When some people think about the act of meditating, they picture some wackadoo sitting in a cross-legged position chanting some undecipherable sounds. Other people have bravely attempted to engage in meditation because someone told them it was a good idea, and they gave up after a minute because it was boring, and they just couldn't sit still. I am about as high energy as they come and, if I can meditate, anyone can meditate.

What is it with this meditation craze? Meditation and mindfulness have been around for centuries and are the fundamental basis of the Buddhist religion. In the past couple of decades, people have started to realize the power that the mind has on the body, and we are revisiting the ancient rituals to gain the serenity that was embraced thousands of years ago.

Have you ever tried so hard to think about something, and it just does not come to you? I know it seems difficult to believe, but we only use a small fraction of our brains. Practically everything that we do every day is a result of some hard-wired connection in our neural circuitry. When you take time to just be, your mind opens up. Neurons that did not communicate in the past start connecting. Heightened creativity and new discoveries come when we put our minds at ease during these moments of solitude. This plays a role in your eye health because when you are creative and productive, you have reduced stress and a healthier mind and body.

Let me now dispel any notion that you cannot meditate. First of all, there are countless ways to meditate, from sitting in one place to taking a walk. You can sit, stand, lay down, or even recline while engaging in this seemingly difficult task. There is no right or wrong way to enter the Zen state of mind.

God, Allah, Buddha—I Don't Care

With the risk of you thinking that I am trying to preach the Bible, I cannot discuss my experience in reversing my eye disease without acknowledging the power that prayer had on my recovery. If not for the moments I spent in prayer, I can almost guarantee that I would not have vision today. God literally directed me onto the path and showed me how to resolve my eye problems. If I heard someone say that, I would think that they are nuts, but, trust me, it happened.

You must understand that I do not care who you consider your higher being. God, Allah, or Buddha, it does not matter. That may offend some people as religion is one of those areas that you are supposed to stay away from, but I just don't care. It would not matter to me if you prayed to a tree or the Earth and considered it your higher power. What is important here is that you connect with something that gives you the ability to reflect, be thankful, visualize, and heal.

When I say reflect, I mean to consider the things in your life that you are happy about and those that weigh heavily on you. You can toss all of these things at whoever it is that you connect with as if you were dumping all of your problems on your best friend. The interesting thing is that as you lay out the things that you feel bad about on this higher power, without the risk of being judged! That is the beauty of prayer! Now, if you told your best friend all of your problems, they might think you are nuts, but not your prayer mate. What's even better is after you lay your thoughts out in prayer, your fears and worries are at ease. So, after three minutes of prayer, you walk out feeling like a new person.

During prayer, you may consider taking a minute to be thankful for everything that you have been given. Even if you feel like your entire world is falling apart, I am sure there is something for which you can give thanks. You will find that if you give more thanks, your stress level goes down. There is always something to appreciate in life. If you ever struggle with what to say or do during a prayer session, I encourage you to start listing the things you are thankful for, and you will feel a sense of happiness within minutes. I pretty much guarantee it!

Perhaps most importantly, prayer heals. There have been numerous attempts to validate the power of prayer through scientific studies. Putting a scientific spin on prayer challenges the essence of faith. The healing that occurs because of prayer is due, at least in part, to the powers of a higher being that are unexplainable. However, if you are an atheist and you just don't resonate with the idea of a higher power, you may consider taking time to reflect and be thankful. The healing power of the mind when you are in a positive mental state is endless.

Now, if the word "prayer" does not resonate with you because it sounds too religious, you can call it a time of thankfulness or simply "me time." What you do during this time is completely up to you. Some ideas for you to consider are journaling, quiet solitude, reading a small passage from your holy book and reflecting on its message, or making a list of things you appreciate.

Journaling may appeal to those people who are intimidated by prayer. When you journal, you simply pick up a pen and paper and write down everything that is heavy on your mind. Moving things from mind to paper aids in the reflection process. Furthermore, when you write what you want and visualize your life, you are more likely to achieve your goals.

As you probably gathered, the *Beyond Carrots* Plan incorporates some version of the prayer that works for you. What will probably surprise you is that I do not care how much time you spend doing this activity. More importantly than the time spent is the consistency of practice. Personally, prayer immediately follows my workout in the morning. What I do during prayer depends on the day and my mood. Occasionally, I will read the Bible and reflect. Other days I will just shoot the breeze with God like he is my friend, and I will ask if my Grandpa Cox and his best friend, Rex, are behaving themselves up there in heaven. (If you ever met my Grandpa Cox, you know the answer to that question is NO!) It does not matter what you talk about; just make time for this powerful activity.

Did You Know Shopping Is Exercise? That Doesn't Sound So Bad, Does It?

If you live in America today, it is hard to avoid hearing about the importance of exercise and its impact on our health. It has been shoved down our throats so much that many people are completely boycotting the exercise bandwagon. What is interesting is how many Americans are overweight and unfit despite the exercise craze.

Although you have heard about the benefits of exercise a million times, let me explain how exercise relates to eye health. The simplest way to explain this connection is to remind you that the entire body is connected. High blood pressure, diabetes, high cholesterol, and stress all negatively impact eye health, as we have discussed throughout this book. The teeny-tiny blood vessels in the eyes are often the first to feel the effects of these diseases. A simple thirty minutes a day of cardiovascular activity can help to reduce each potentially vision-threatening disease.

Your eye is an extension of your brain. In other words, exercise also impacts your brain and can reduce your risk of developing Alzheimer's and dementia. You could go so far as to say that time spent exercising makes you smarter.

If your reason for not working out is that you just don't have enough time, let me tell you something interesting. Working out can increase productivity and energy levels so that you can get more done in less time. Exercise even improves sleep quality. Exercise is considered a keystone habit, so when you ritualize a morning workout routine, you are more likely to go to bed at a reasonable time and wake up refreshed and ready to get in that workout.

As far as which type of exercise is best, quite frankly, whatever makes you motivated to move is the best form of exercise for you. For instance, my mom is an avid shopper and would walk twenty miles a day if it meant she could shop. Whether you call it taking a walk or spending money, it gets the body moving, and that is what matters the most. On the other hand, I love the feeling of a brisk swim as I watch the sunrise through the South Florida palm trees, so taking a dip in the pool first thing is my exercise of choice. Heck, you can even crunch out some curls and binge-watch Netflix at the same time! If you already have some sort of routine in place and are looking to take your fitness to the next level, there is some solid research around the benefits of high-intensity interval training and its benefits on the cardiovascular system and calorie burning.

In my opinion, the biggest challenge to working out is deciding to work out and determining a workout routine. To make this easier, I would recommend that you decide at the start of the week what day and time you are going to squeeze in some movement. Choosing to do your physical training first thing in the morning is always best so you can get it done before the day gets the best of you. Set out all the equipment that you will need for your exercise the night before. I would even advise that you set out your clothes and shoes to minimize thinking in the morning. If you are doing a workout online, have the workout at the tip of your fingers, so you have minimal effort when you wake up.

Now, here is the trick. When your alarm goes off, tell yourself that you are going to do just five minutes of your workout, and then you can go back to bed. If you finish five minutes of your workout and truly want to go back to sleep, go for it! I highly doubt that will happen. A body in motion stays in motion. You will find that as soon as you start moving, your day feels more amazing, and your energy level stays elevated!

In the *Beyond Carrots* Plan, we will walk through a plan for determining what you need to do to get your butt moving. This will require thinking out of the box, especially if you are not already driven to hit the gym. I will help you figure out what will get you in better shape than you have been in years. This is not a one size fits all plan, but I promise you will be the happiest you have ever been when you put this plan into place. So, let's get moving!

Vitamin D vs. UV Light

There is nothing I love more than dichotomy because, without it, life would be boring. If you are wondering what dichotomy I am talking about, sunlight is a dichotomous entity. It is potentially toxic and vitalizing at the same time. How funny is it that we wake up and feel invigorated when we see the sunrise, yet we need sunblock to fend our bodies from its damaging rays? Not enough sunlight can bring you to a state of deep depression, but too much light can cause blindness. So, what do we need to do to reap the benefits of this magical ball of fire without putting ourselves in danger? The research has shown that ultraviolet rays can damage every square inch of your body, and your eyes are no exception. So, let's break down eye problems associated with UV light, starting with the outer part of the eye.

What Eye Conditions Result from the Damaging Rays of UV Light?

Many people who have worked outside without sunglasses develops a sort of yellow lump on either the white part of the eye or the cornea. This callus can become red and inflamed when the eyes are extremely dry. The affected area is called either a pinguecula or a pterygium, depending on whether it affects the white part of the eye or the cornea, respectively. Wearing sunglasses dramatically reduces your risk of developing this condition. However, if the damaged area gets big enough, you and your doctor can talk about surgery as an option.

When sunlight hits the lens of the eye, it causes immediate destruction. As a result, the proteins of the lens become all messed up, and you get cataract formation. Quite frankly, cataracts are going to come at some point in time, whether you wear sunglasses or not, so brace yourself for this reality. Protective eyewear will certainly slow the progression of the lens changes that can account for more vision loss worldwide than any other eye problem. In America, we are quite fortunate to have health care at our fingertips and surgery options to remove these pesky cataracts easily.

Moving along to the back part of the eye, we find the retina that contains the nerves for light perception. If you have ever seen a fire start by holding a magnifying glass reflecting sunlight on a piece of paper, you can imagine what sunlight does to the back part of the eye. Your retina is constantly trying to clean up the destruction created by these UV rays, but, occasionally, blindness can result from your body's inability to protect itself from the rays of the sun. This is the case in macular degeneration, where the best central vision part of the retina faces extreme damage due to a number of factors. Sunlight is one of the elements that contribute to the development of this potentially sight-threatening condition.

What Benefits Does Sunlight Have on Our Bodies and Eyes?

In sharp contrast to the sun's damaging effects on every square inch of our bodies, the sun is critical for our survival. Sunlight contributes to our bodies' production of vitamin D, but it is very difficult to get all of the vitamin D that our bodies need from the sun alone. There are a handful of foods that contain vitamin D ranging from salmon and sardines to egg yolk. However, in general, most of the vitamin D we consume in our foods is fortified, as you see in milk and yogurt. For some people, it may be necessary to supplement with vitamin D tablets. Before you start popping vitamin D pills, I recommend that you get some baseline blood work done to know where you stand right now. We will dive into baseline testing when we discuss the *Beyond Carrots* Plan.

Why is Vitamin D so Important?

Vitamin D aids every square inch of our bodies. It helps regulate our bodies' absorption of minerals like calcium and phosphorous, which helps to keep our bones and muscles strong. Vitamin D also supports our immune system by fighting off infections like the cold and flu. Even more, it helps prevent autoimmune attacks, as you see in multiple sclerosis and cardiovascular disease.

If that is not enough for you to get your vitamin D levels checked, let's talk about the effects that vitamin D can have on your mind. Studies show that low vitamin D levels can contribute to depression, Alzheimer's, and dementia. Now you see why vitamin D is so important that it made it into our shortlist of vitamins in the KISS vitamin part of the *Beyond Carrots* Plan.

Get Those Zzz's

Of all the lifestyle hacks we will address, sleep is, perhaps, the most important. Getting too little or too much sleep can have detrimental effects on our bodies and contribute to vision loss. We will discuss many of the diseases and potential eye problems that can result from poor sleep schedules. If you are one of the many people who have a difficult time falling asleep and staying asleep, I will give you some simple tips that are sure to put you into a restful state and keep you there.

Pretty much every system of your body is affected by sleep. To be clear, we are shooting for seven to eight hours of good quality sleep per night. Sleeping less than six and over ten hours can increase the likelihood of acquiring diabetes, high blood pressure, and other cardiovascular diseases. If that's not enough, your risk of becoming obese increases dramatically when you either oversleep or under sleep. Have you ever noticed that you catch a common cold when you go a couple of nights with minimum sleep? Well, it should not surprise you that your immune system weakens when you skip out on those Zs. We are just scraping the surface of all the effects that sleep can have on your body.

The most well-known eye problem that is linked to a sleeping disorder is floppy eyelid syndrome and sleep apnea. An overwhelming percentage of those people with sleep apnea also have a condition known as floppy eyelid syndrome, where the eyelid is weak. This condition results in lids that flop around like untoned belly fat, so it got the name floppy eyelid syndrome. I mention this connection to show how a sleep disorder can affect your eyes, but this is just one example. I promise, there is more to come.

What is the first thing you notice when you wake up and look in the mirror after a sleepless night? Wow . . . my eyes look and feel terrible! They probably look red with heavy lids, and they feel dry and scratchy. Too little sleep contributes to dry eye syndrome, a condition we discussed earlier. Dry eye syndrome contributes to depression and results in psychological frustration, which can further complicate your sleep hygiene. It becomes a vicious cycle that will perpetually complicate your life and your health.

Too much sleep can be equally destructive to your eye health. In fact, research shows that sleeping over eight hours a night can contribute to the dry form of age-related macular degeneration. It is important to note here that too much of a good thing is no longer a good thing. So, do not try to oversleep thinking that you are going to be super healthy because that is not the way it works. Try to keep your sleep between the recommended seven to nine hours of sleep with a goal of a solid eight.

The most compelling research around sleep and eye health is around glaucoma, a potentially blinding eye disease. You are three times more likely to get glaucoma when you sleep less than three hours or over ten hours a night. So that's a pretty good reason to keep your sleep in the recommended time frame and avoid excess sleeping.

So many people talk about how difficult it is for them to go to sleep and stay asleep. I am going to give you some simple suggestions that, when implemented, are sure to help improve your sleep quality and elevate your mood. By creating nightly routines that incorporate healthy habits, you can improve every aspect of your life.

First and foremost, figure out a set bedtime and stick to it. Try to go to sleep and get up within thirty minutes of your set time each and every day. You may want to make your bedtime 10 p.m. and your wake time 6 a.m. It does not matter what time you choose. What matters most is that you do not deviate from this time. If you keep a schedule for long enough, your body will start to remember what time you are supposed to go to sleep and will naturally get sleepy at that time.

I cannot overemphasize the importance of exercising to improve sleep hygiene. When you exercise, your stress hormones decrease, and your happy hormones increase. I am simplifying this, but the main point here is that thirty minutes of moderate-intensity cardiovascular movement daily will improve your sleep quality, and you will be a happier person.

Believe it or not, sunlight can dramatically impact sleep patterns. Your eyes see the sunlight, and hormones are released, telling you it is time to wake up and get things done. Likewise, darkness promotes the sleepy time hormones, and you enter a more restful state. To promote this sleep/wake cycle that is better known as your circadian rhythm, you should shoot for a minimum of thirty minutes a day with some direct daylight exposure.

There are two main reasons why this is effective at reducing stress and increasing sleep quality. First of all, enjoying nature will reduce your stress hormones and will result in better sleep. Even if you do not have time to go to a nature preserve daily, simply enjoying the outdoors by watching a bird fly outside your office building will help to reduce your stress. Secondly, the sunlight you are exposed to will rejuvenate you and help remind your body that it is daytime and time to expend every last bit of energy. This way, when the lights go out at night, you are sure to hit the sack like a ton of bricks.

Along the same lines, I would strongly recommend one solid hour of absolutely no technology preceding your determined bedtime. I know that seems like it is next to impossible as you need your phone to function at all times of the day, but you can do it! This simple habit of limiting technology will put your mind and body at ease and simplify the transition from the constant movement of your mind during the day to the state of restfulness that puts you to sleep. Try limiting technology for ten days and see how you feel. I have a feeling you are going to be astonished at how much better you sleep, and you are going to learn to love your technology-free time.

Smartphones, computers, and tablets shoot bright lights into our eyes. In the medical world, we call the light that comes out of these devices blue light. In the past couple of years, blue light has gotten much more attention as it is potentially damaging to the back part of the eye. Furthermore, blue light confuses the body into thinking it is still daytime because the lights are so bright. So, when you are staring at your computer, phone, or iPad until 10 p.m. and then try to go to sleep, your brain is super confused, and it is much more difficult to get yourself to your slumber state. Just try to limit your device use and see how you feel!

There are a couple of tips on beverages of choice to promote healthy sleep patterns. It should come as no surprise that you should try to limit coffee and caffeine during the second half of the day as it can interfere with sleep. As for alcohol, it may feel like a glass of wine or two will put you right to sleep, but alcohol negatively impacts your sleep quality. Although you may be able to get to sleep faster, the quality of sleep will suffer. I would recommend considering replacing your glass of wine with a cup of warm, cozy chamomile tea that is sure to put you to sleep.

Believe it or not, certain foods can help to put you to sleep because they contain a hormone called melatonin. Specifically, tart cherries and almonds are two such foods that, when eaten in the evening, can help get your body and mind ready for a full eight hours of blissful sleep. Give a bowl of tart cherries and almonds a shot, you have got nothing to lose, and they sure do taste good together!

There are a couple of things that you may consider doing during your technology-free hour that are super relaxing and sleep-promoting. Light stretching in bed or on the floor of a dark room feels amazing and helps get your mind off the day and into sleep mode. Alternatively, you may want to take a warm bath with lavender aromatherapy during your technology-free time if you want to do nothing for a minute. The magic of the calming water and scents of lavender is sure to calm every bone in your body.

The goal here is to develop daytime habits and an evening routine that facilitates your ability to get seven to eight hours of good quality sleep daily. You will find that you have more energy and improved overall health when you make these changes. I would go so far as to say that this is one of the most important aspects of the *Beyond Carrots* Plan as changing habits around sleep trickle down to impact every area of your life.

It is Long, White, Skinny, and Kills Just About Every Bone in Your Body

When I started to write about smoking, I thought about all the "STOP SMOKING" campaigns that have been going on for years. You have to be living in a box to think that smoking is not damaging to your body. If millions of dollars in government money to educate the public on the damaging effects of smoking does not work, what makes me think that my input will help? My goal here is to give you some practical tips to consider that may be slightly different than other options. I also hope to congratulate those people who have made the accomplishment of omitting smoking from their lives. Lastly, for those individuals who are on the verge of vision loss yet still smoking, I hope to educate you on the effects that those little devils have on your eyes to get you to join the smoke-free bandwagon. It is never too late to escape the cigarette prison.

I am going to give you a very simplified view of why smoking is bad for your body and eyes. Every day, our trusty old body faces mini-battles against little things that we encounter during the day. For instance, the sun hits our skin and eyes, and the body has to fight off the toxic effects of the sun. You may scrape your knee, and the body needs to try to heal that wound. You may eat a half dozen Krispy Kreme donuts for lunch, and your digestive tract goes into toxin overload. (PS, if you think it is impossible to eat a half dozen Krispy Kremes, I suggest you hang out with my mom for the day!) In any case, there are so many minor attacks that the body faces daily and is usually able to handle on an individual basis.

When you smoke a cigarette, it is like an atomic bomb explodes in the lungs that quickly migrates throughout the body, into the nervous system and bloodstream. Your body cannot begin to fight off the toxins from the sun or deal with the Krispy Kreme donuts when it is trying to defend itself from the offenders that just entered the body with the smoke that was inhaled. The body throws its immune defense system into overdrive to deal with the cigarette bomb. We all know what happens when this system is overworked. That's right—disease!

Perhaps the most well-recognized eye disease that results from smoking is macular degeneration. Cataracts also come on much earlier for a smoker because the eye's lens needs to fight the toxins in the body and cannot maintain its own clarity. If you have ever looked at a smoker's eyes, you may notice that they are less white and sometimes red and irritated. Smoking contributes to dry eye syndrome because the lacrimal gland reduces its tear production. As if that is not enough, the smoker has to contend with the fact that cancer can actually spread to the eye. Malignant melanoma in the eye is grounds for enucleation, a procedure when the entire eyeball is removed.

Even though smokers have been told over and over again the importance of putting the cigarette down, quitting is extremely difficult. There is a chemical and habitual addiction to the nasty habit. I would like to think that I have the magic bullet to help you quit, but I don't. I can, however, give you some helpful hints on how to manage the habit.

It only makes sense to reduce the stress in your life because your willpower to change a habit dwindles quickly when you are stressed out. I know, reducing stress in your life is not as simple as it sounds. I am right there in the trenches with all of you! Anything you can do to reduce stress in your life is a step in the right direction.

The second aspect to consider when trying to quit smoking is that smoking is a habit. Habits are ingrained into our neuropathways so much that we automatically reach for the cigarette at various times of the day or as we do certain activities. The good news is that neuropathways are modifiable. You can relearn associations with various tasks. It may sound crazy, but hypnosis is actually an excellent way to retrain your brain on the most subconscious level.

Although I have never been a smoker, I can only imagine how difficult it must be to quit such an addictive habit. I can remember my grandpa asking for a cigarette in the hospital on the day he died from lung cancer. It broke my heart to watch him die, and I pray that I can help just one person avoid his terrible suffering.

Chapter 6:

Beyond Carrots Plan

The Two *Beyond Carrots* Plans

Let me tell you what happened when I created the *Beyond Carrots* Plan. I outlined what foods you should eat and avoid to reverse eye disease and revitalize your body. This information is based on my extensive research, education as an Anti-Aging Health Practitioner, and my personal experience. Many people have asked me how I reversed my eye disease, so I shared my exact regimen. I also discussed the lifestyle changes that may seem insignificant but truly played into your plan's success.

When I finished writing my plan, I was ecstatic to finally document how people could follow in my footpath and change their vision's fate. I got over my excitement when I reread the plan, only to realize that my plan was super labor-intensive and required an incredible amount of determination. This posed a big problem because if my plan was too difficult to execute, many readers might say forget it. For the people who decided to try to execute my original plan, the amount of willpower required to sustain the *Beyond Carrots* Plan could only last so long. I was afraid that upon the completion of the first thirty days, my readers would end up reverting to their same old habits.

With those considerations in mind, I created the "Baby Steps *Beyond Carrots* Plan." The Baby Steps *Beyond Carrots* Plan is meant to be a guide in creating changes in diet and lifestyle that will last a lifetime. This plan aims to make small changes every month to the foods you eat and the lifestyle choices you make so that you have made twelve alterations to your life that will help create a healthier version of you at the end of a year.

Nonetheless, I would recommend that everyone read the entire *Beyond Carrots* Plan, which is full of important information. When you finish reading the plan, you can decide what group of people you fall into. If you are faced with a potentially blinding eye disease or life-threatening medical condition, and you are as scared as I was that you may never be able to see again, you will have the drive to execute the original plan. However, if you are reading this book because you feel pretty good but would like to reduce your chances of experiencing vision loss, I recommend you embrace the "Baby Steps *Beyond Carrots* Plan." When you put this modified plan into action, no matter how small the change may seem, you will see improvements that will motivate you to continue to move forward.

Beyond Carrots Plan, Step 1: Mentally Prepare

Anytime you set out to accomplish something, you must set an intention for what you want to achieve. This is, perhaps, the most important step in the *Beyond Carrots* Plan and will require some time, so please do not take this step lightly. Our goal is to create a clear and concise mission statement that reflects your values and make that statement a part of your daily life.

Before you begin, get yourself a lined spiral notebook and write on the front of it, *Beyond Carrots* Plan. You want to write down goals, take baseline readings, and track progress. Writing things down is at the core of the *Beyond Carrots* Plan. If you do not write it down, you will lose direction and will have no way of knowing where you are and where you started. Documentation also improves accountability because when you can track progress, you will be more likely to stay on track.

Next, take a minute to think about what it is that you value most in life. What is it that is at the core of everything that you do? What makes you smile? How do you define yourself? Some of the values that you may consider are the following:

- Loyalty
- Good humor
- Open-mindedness
- Honesty
- Spirituality
- Passion
- Respect
- Fitness
- Family
- Courage
- Perseverance
- Education
- Community service
- Adventure
- Patriotism
- Optimism
- Consistency
- Love

This is just a short list to get you thinking about what makes you tick and drives your every action. After you have put some thought into these questions, please write down on the first page of your *Beyond Carrots* notebook three to five values that are at the core of every decision that you make in life. This will be the foundation on which we build YOUR *Beyond Carrots* Plan.

Next, think about your overall objectives in your *Beyond Carrots* journey. You should create one to three objectives that align with the core values that you just wrote down. We want to stay laser-focused on the goals of your journey; having more than three objectives can be overwhelming. By the way, these objectives do not necessarily have to do with improving eye health. For example, you may want to reduce your blood sugar level or reduce arthritic pains. By following the *Beyond Carrots* Plan, you will reduce inflammation across your body, ease the strain on your hand and wrist, and improve eye health all at the same time! Another person's objective may be to lose ten pounds. Although the *Beyond Carrots* Plan is not specifically aimed towards weight loss, you have the potential to lose weight by following this guide. Believe it or not, as you get closer to your ideal weight, you will improve your eye health.

After you have one to three clear objectives, take a moment to consider the time frame in which you would like to accomplish these tasks. For instance, if you have had severe pain in your hand and wrist for years, you may want to give yourself three months to see a reverse in your discomfort. On the other hand, if you have your son's wedding in three months and want to be ten pounds lighter on the day of his wedding, then you would make your son's wedding date the target date to keep in mind. The main point here is that you must have a clearly delineated target date for a goal; otherwise, you lose focus.

Now we need to pull it all together by writing a mission statement. The mission statement should be written in the following format, "In my *Beyond Carrots* journey, I will [insert objective] by [target date] because I [core value]." For instance, when I started my *Beyond Carrots* journey, my mission statement was, "I will reverse my potentially blinding eye disease in thirty days because I value my health." You should create similar mission statements for each objective.

Your mission statement that we just created does no good for your written in a notebook that you do not see daily. You must have your mission statement in plain sight daily to be constantly reminded of where you are going. You know you better than I know you, so put your statement wherever you will see it. One idea for you to consider is putting your statement on a small corkboard surrounded by pictures that exemplify your vision of what you will look and feel like when you accomplish your objective. A fancy word for this corkboard is a vision board. This board can be as simple or as complex as you would like. What is most important is that it is visible daily.

The purpose of this process is to help you hone in on your values and give you a laser-sharp picture of where we are going together on this journey. This may take one person one hour and another individual one week. It does not matter how long it takes you to write your statement. Just make it happen in order to have a solid base on which to build your *Beyond Carrots* Plan.

Beyond Carrots Plan, Step 2: Baseline Testing

Let's say that you were going on a road trip from Florida to California. The first thing that you would need to do is your exact starting point. The same holds for the *Beyond Carrots* journey. Before you dive into fixing your mind, body, and eyes, you must get information about what is going on in your body at this time. This information will act as a baseline so that you can easily measure your improvement as you execute every step of the *Beyond Carrots* Plan. I will promise you at least one of these baseline measurements will improve if you follow this plan exactly.

I would like to reiterate that this is designed to reverse eye disease; however, it is not exclusively intended for those facing possible vision loss. The ultimate purpose of the *Beyond Carrots* Plan is to improve the health of your body, mind, and eyes. I assure you, with a healthy body and mind come healthy eyes.

The first appointment that you need to make when doing baseline testing is with, that's right, your eye doctor! The most important part of your visit with the eye doctor is the eye health evaluation so, please, do not skip the assessment of the back part of the eyes. Your doctor should complete a full eye exam and will collect a plethora of information. For the purposes of our baseline testing, please obtain the following information from your physician upon the completion of your eye exam:

1. Visual acuity with and without glasses
2. Glasses prescription
3. Schirmer's test
4. Eye health evaluation: slit lamp exam and retina evaluation
5. Ocular coherence tomography (OCT) (if available)
6. Contrast sensitivity (if available)
7. Macular Pigment Ocular Density (MPOD) (if available)

Visual Acuity With and Without Glasses

We will break down each of the items you will gather on your trip to the eye doctor. The first item on this list measures the level of your vision without glasses measured one eye at a time. This measurement is usually written as 20/X. You interpret this reading by saying that you can see at twenty feet what the person with perfect vision can see at X feet. So, if your vision is 20/40, that would mean that you have to go up to twenty feet to see what the person with perfect vision can see at forty feet. In other words, when the second number is lower, you have better vision. This visual acuity reading should be measured with and without glasses in anticipation of possible improvement of the visual acuity as you carry out your *Beyond Carrots* Plan.

Glasses Prescription

It is also important to document your glasses prescription at the start of your *Beyond Carrots* journey. We may find that as you lose weight and get your health under control, you may find a shift in your glasses prescription. Our ultimate goal is to improve the actual visual acuity but keeping an eye on the actual prescription in your glasses is a good idea.

Schirmer's Test

Most optometrists can do a Schirmer's test to measure the level your level of eye dryness. This test uses a small strip of paper placed next to the lid. The doctor measure how many tears gather on the piece of paper to help grade your level of dry eye. Ideally, you would get a level between eight and ten millimeters of wetting. Through the *Beyond Carrots* Plan, we aim to reduce ocular inflammation and increase eye moisture.

Eye Health Evaluation: Slit Lamp Exam and Retina Evaluation

The eye health evaluation is, perhaps, the most important part of your visit with the eye doctor. The slit lamp exam allows the doctor to take a close look at the front part of the eye using a thin beam of light and the retina evaluation is a health evaluation of the back part of the eye. I will say it over and over again, "You can have perfect eyes and still have a blinding eye disease, so do not skip your retina evaluation." Photodocumentation is the best form of documentation, and the newest widefield cameras give amazing photos. In my practices, we use the newest technology in widefield photos to completely evaluate the retina. Even though dilation is the standard of care for all first-time patients, I feel that I am doing a disservice by not using widefield photodocumentation to assess eye health completely. Be sure to document any abnormalities while performing the health assessment in one of your *Beyond Carrots* resources.

Ocular Coherence Tomography (OCT) (if available)

To get an even better assessment of every layer of the back part of the eye, consider getting an OCT if that is available at your eye doctor's office. The OCT is a quick scan of the retina and optic nerve that helps to find macular degeneration, glaucoma, and other diseases before they are visible by the naked eye with the retina camera. This test takes no more than two minutes and does not require any eye drops.

Contrast Sensitivity and MPOD (if available)

The last two items on our list, contrast sensitivity and MPOD testing, are not routinely performed during an eye exam. Not all doctors can do these tests, and they may be next to impossible for you to include in your assessment. I mention these additional tests because they are fantastic indicators of your eyesight improvement as you work your way through the *Beyond Carrots* Plan.

Contrast sensitivity measures how well you see in low contrast situations and is a great indicator of your eye health. This test is performed by reading the eye chart with various levels of grayscale in the letters seen. The results are given as a percentage number. One would predict that your contrast sensitivity score would improve as you improve your mind, body, and eyes by executing the steps in the *Beyond Carrots* Plan. If you can find a doctor with this test, great! Otherwise, don't sweat it.

An even more difficult test for you to get your hands on at an eye doctor's office is the macular pigment ocular density test (MPOD). This test tells us about the amount of pigment and antioxidants accumulated at the best central vision part of the back part of the eye. This test is non-invasive and involves a quick scan of the eyeball. The results are given on a scale from 0 to 1. MPOD results from 0 to 0.21 are low, 0.21 to 0.44 are midrange, and 0.44 to 1 are high. One of the main goals of the *Beyond Carrots* Plan is to increase the antioxidant levels throughout the body. This would result in higher MPOD scores and healthier eyes.

Next, you will get a series of blood tests done using an order from your eye doctor or medical doctor. If your eye doctor has connections with a lab that can run blood tests, you can bring the following tests to the eye doctor and request the tests to be performed. If the eye doctor cannot communicate with a blood lab, you can bring the following list with you to your medical doctor or nurse practitioner to write up the order.

1. Inflammatory markers: C-reactive protein (CRP) and erythrocyte sedimentation rate (ESR)
2. Blood sugar levels: Hba1C and fasting blood sugar level
3. Cholesterol
4. Blood pressure
5. Vitamin D, specifically 1.25-dihydroxy vitamin D
6. Fish oil: EPA and DHA in the blood

You should discuss the results of each of the tests performed above with the ordering physician or nurse practitioner. You should also document in your *Beyond Carrots* notebook the results of these five tests. I will provide some general information to explain why these tests are important to perform. Still, your physician is ultimately in charge of deciding on an action plan upon completing your bloodwork.

Inflammatory Markers

Inflammatory markers are items that are tested for in the blood that indicate if you inflammation in any part of your body. The tricky thing about inflammatory markers is you may have normal test results when you do the bloodwork for these markers but still have low-grade inflammation. So, although it is very important to get this information before we begin our journey together, you are not necessarily inflammation-free if your test results come back normal. The two inflammatory markers that I am focusing on are C-reactive protein and erythrocyte sedimentation rate. Because labs can vary slightly in the range for normal versus abnormal test results, I will defer the interpretation of the results of these tests to your physician. All I want you to do is to document your test results in your *Beyond Carrots* notebook so that we can monitor for change.

Blood Sugar Levels

For your *Beyond Carrots* Plan, the second category of testing that should be done when you go to your physician is a blood sugar level evaluation. You should have this test done to ensure that you are not diabetic or borderline diabetic. The newest research shows that nearly a third of all Americans have diabetes and are unaware of their disease. You must always follow the guidance of your medical doctor when you find the results of the blood sugar evaluation.

One of the many goals of the *Beyond Carrots* Plan is to help control blood sugar without medication. Diabetes can wreak havoc on the back part of the eye, and a few simple modifications to your daily routine can help lower your blood sugar and reduce the need for medications. Simply document the results of these tests in your spiral notebook, so we know where you are starting.

Cholesterol

While they are poking you for everything else, make sure that they check your cholesterol levels. It is a good idea to have your cholesterol levels evaluated, but do not freak out if you get an abnormal result. Your cholesterol level can fluctuate significantly based on the food you eat, physical activity, and hormones. Seasonal variations can even affect cholesterol levels. I would like for you to make a note of where you are starting so that we have some point of reference. You must always follow the advice of your medical doctor, but through the *Beyond Carrots* Plan, we hope to see a reduction in your cholesterol level.

Blood Pressure

Blood pressure is another item that can go up or down fairly significantly; just ask my mom. She says that any time I hang out with my friends in Fort Lauderdale, her blood pressure goes through the roof. I don't blame her—I have my wild moments! Consistently high blood pressure is a big problem on pretty much every organ in your body, including your eyeballs. Document where you are, and as always, follow the medical recommendations from your physician. If your blood pressure is elevated, it is our goal to naturally lower your blood pressure to the point where, hopefully, you won't need blood pressure medications. I know this sounds impossible, but I truly believe that we got this!

Vitamin D Levels

You will find out when we get to the KISS vitamin chapter that I am not a huge fan of taking a ton of vitamins. Vitamin D is one of the few vitamins that I feel is very important to get tested for and supplement when necessary. The aspects of your health that vitamin D affects are limitless. Vitamin D affects bone production, energy levels, mood, wound healing, and the immune system. Low vitamin D levels can contribute to dementia, osteoporosis, and overall body discomfort. The good news is that it is very easy to access vitamin D supplementation; improving deficiency in this vitamin will occur throughout our time together. Document, document, document! We have to know where you are starting so that we can smile when we see improvement.

Blood EPA/DHA Levels

The last test that we would complete in our little ideal world would be a test for the amount of fish oil in your blood. Not all doctors can test for this level, as there are a select few labs that can run this test. Most functional medicine physicians have access to special labs that can run this test for you. You are testing for the level of EPA (eicosapentaenoic acid) and DHA (docosahexaenoic acid) in the blood. EPA and DHA are two components of fish oil whose levels in our bodies are measurable through bloodwork. Most people have low levels of EPA and DHA, which affects everything from the heart and brain to the eyes and immune system. I am pretty sure that you will see some improvement in your fish oil levels with the implementation of this program.

Lastly, we have a couple of things to do at home along the lines of baseline testing:
1. Measure your body weight.
2. Determine your BMI.
3. Measure waist circumference.

4. Measure bowel transit time after eating one cup of beets.
5. Complete the Perceived Stress Scale Test to get a numerical number that indicates your current stress level.
6. Complete the *Beyond Carrots* Inflammatory Questionnaire to get a numerical measurement of the inflammatory symptoms that you are currently experiencing.

Body Weight

Although our main purpose in the *Beyond Carrots* Plan is to reverse eye disease, you may notice weight loss in the process. Your body weight should be measured first thing in the morning after you use the restroom and before you eat. As you know from our discussion of the Three Stooges, diabetes, high blood pressure, and obesity are three compounding diseases that can contribute to eye disease. Therefore, getting weight under control is a must if you are looking to reduce the risk of going blind.

Body Mass Index

Your BMI is determined using two measurements, your height and your weight. This number has increasingly become the gold standard measurement to determine if you are underweight, overweight, or normal weight. Different studies have varying numbers on the exact range for the ideal BMI. In general, if your BMI is lower than 18.5, you are considered underweight, and if your BMI is over 25, you are considered overweight. The further you are from this ideal range, the higher risk you have for dying early. I think that is a pretty good reason to know your BMI!

You can calculate this number by taking your weight in pounds and dividing it by your height in inches squared and multiplying by 703.

$$BMI = \left[\frac{weight\ in\ pounds}{(height\ in\ inches)^2}\right] * 703$$

Waist Circumference

As you lose weight, you will likely notice a reduction in your waist circumference. It is important to document your waist circumference because, in cases where there is muscle growth, you may see that your weight does not change even though your waist circumference decreases. If you are on the thin side, you may find your waist circumference increases as you increase your intake of nutritious foods. We want to be able to track this progress in your journey. Your waist circumference should be taken using a cloth tape measure that you wrap all the way around your tummy at the level of your belly button.

Bowel Transit Time

The next thing that we are going to do as part of your homework is measure how fast something moves from your mouth to your butt, otherwise known as bowel transit time. A simple way to take this measurement is to eat a half-cup to a cup of beets. If you are pooping red in 12–24 hours, you are doing great! If your poop is red in less than twelve hours, you probably have malabsorption of nutrients. The most common problem is that it takes way too long for the poop to turn red from the beets that you had for lunch. If your transit time is over twenty-four hours, then it is possible that toxins are not being eliminated quickly enough by your digestive system. As part of the *Beyond Carrots* Plan, we will be freshening up the digestive system and healing the gut with probiotics and prebiotics that may have an impact on this bowel transit time.

Stress Level

There is probably not a single person reading this book that can tell me they have no stress in their life. Stress is inevitable and difficult to measure precisely. For the purposes of the *Beyond Carrots* Plan, we are using a well-recognized perceived stress test to get a numerical measurement of how much stress you have in your life before beginning our journey together. Through the simple steps outlined in this plan and the support in the *Beyond Carrots* community, we expect to see a reduction in your level of perceived stress. Print out the Perceived Stress Scale Test using link below or access on the resource page of the Beyond Carrots website, www.beyondcarrots.com, and perform the simple ten-question test coming up with a numerical score that you record in your notebook. If all goes as planned, that number will be lower with the help of *Beyond Carrots*.

https://das.nh.gov/wellness/Docs/Percieved%20Stress%20Scale.pdf

Beyond Carrots Inflammatory Questionnaire

Last but not least, complete the following *Beyond Carrots* Inflammatory Questionnaire. You will find a list of symptoms that you will rank on a scale from zero to five. Add up your score to get a numerical measurement of your level of discomfort due to your inflammatory disease. Assessing these symptoms is important because inflammation is not localized to one part of your body. As we reverse the inflammation in your eyes, we may see a reduction in inflammation throughout the body. We must document the severity of your symptoms before we dive into this *Beyond Carrots* adventure.

Inflammatory Questionnaire

Please rank on a scale from 0–5 (zero indicating never, and five indicating always). Then add up the numbers to get your total score.

Eyes
_____How often do you notice that your eyes are red or irritated?
_____How often do you notice that your eyes are dry?
_____How often do you notice pain or discomfort around the eyes?
_____How often do you get headaches?
_____How often do you get bumps on your eyelid?
_____How often do you notice that your vision gets blurry?

Skin/Hair/Nails
_____How often do you notice that your skin is flaking?
_____How often do you notice that you get acne?
_____How often do you notice that your hair is falling out?
_____How often do you notice that your nails are getting thinner and breaking easily?

Neurologic System
_____How often do you find yourself getting up in the middle of the night because you are unable to sleep?
_____How often do you find yourself losing attention easily?

_____How often do you notice that you have a poor memory?
_____How often do you get migraines?

Mood and Emotions
_____How often do you experience depression or anxiety?
_____How often do you find yourself experiencing excessive mood swings?
_____How often do you find yourself extremely lethargic?

Digestive System
_____How often do you find that you are constipated?
_____How often do you find that you have diarrhea?
_____How often do you find yourself bloated?
_____How often do you experience heartburn or indigestion?
_____How often do you get cancer sores around your mouth?
_____How often do you notice your mouth is excessively dry?
_____How often do you get food cravings?
_____How difficult is it for you to maintain the ideal weight?

Heart and Lungs
_____How often do you notice you are short of breath?
_____How often do you get chest congestion?
_____How often is your heartbeat irregular?
_____How often do you get discomfort in or around your chest?

_____TOTAL SCORE

Document this total score in your *Beyond Carrots* notebook. By implementing this system, we hope to revisit this questionnaire and find that your score has decreased. However, even if we find a small decrease in the score on this test, we are on the right track.

Beyond Carrots Plan, Step 3: Spring Cleaning

There is something about getting junk out of the house that is so much fun! Well, it is spring cleaning time for all of us, and we are going to focus on removing anything at all that can cause inflammation in any part of our bodies. Every person reading this book is likely to have some level of inflammation in your body. Our aim here is to eliminate those things from your life that may be contributing to your inflammation.

Some of the foods that we will be eliminating are toxic and should not be reintroduced to your diet at any time. Other foods that we will be discussing are potentially pro-inflammatory to some people and should be set aside temporarily as we work on healing your body. When you get yourself to a point where you are feeling better and your test results are to a level where you and your physician are happy, you can slowly reintroduce foods one food at a time. We are taking it slowly here because if something triggers your immune system and makes you uncomfortable, we need to nip it in the bud.

The good news is that I will keep the list of clearly toxic foods nice and short. The list of things that I want you to focus on avoiding permanently includes refined sugar and processed foods. That sounds simple, right? The problem is that sugar is everywhere! Sodas, breads, potato chips, many types of cookies, some jarred tomato sauces, and candy are all packed with refined sugar that are terrible for every bone in our bodies. Likewise, processed foods run rampant through the grocery aisles. Some lunch meat, hot dogs, cereal, cheeses, and lots of things in a box are all processed and destroy our bodies, brains, and eyes.

The list of potentially problematic foods that we will temporarily set aside and reintroduce to our diet slowly includes gluten, nightshades, legumes, eggs, coffee, and alcohol. Wait, did I say *alcohol*? I am not telling you to give up alcohol forever. I would never say that. We just need to set the beer, wine, and gin and tonic aside for a short time as we heal our bodies as they are all foods that can exacerbate problems in our gut and immune system. If I can give up alcohol for a period of time, you can too!

Did I also sneak coffee into that shortlist of foods to temporarily set aside? I am so sneaky, aren't I? Coffee has tons of great health benefits, and I would not recommend discontinuing coffee forever. I would, however, slowly cut back on coffee to the point where you have eliminated coffee from your diet. If you are starting at two cups per day, drink one cup a day for a week, then half a cup a day for a week, then stop coffee altogether. You see, the problem with coffee is that it can contribute to inflammation, and it can irritate the gut. We really want to eliminate all chances that we have any form of inflammation in our bodies, so we should give the coffee a break.

You may notice that this list of potentially problematic foods includes eggs, legumes, and nightshades. Yes, I know; I told you a bit ago that these foods are very nutrient-dense and fantastic for the eyes. Because these foods can wreak havoc in some people's bodies and ramp up their autoimmune diseases, it is best to set them aside temporarily and look for other sources of nutrient-dense foods.

The goal of the *Beyond Carrots* Plan is to heal the body to the point that we can make sure that inflammation is to a minimum. If you are asymptomatic and going through the *Beyond Carrots* Plan to ensure you have the healthiest eyes possible, you should maintain this regimen of toxin elimination for thirty days. If you have one or more areas of your body or eyes that is suffering from some sort of disease, you should keep these potentially damaging foods eliminated for sixty to ninety days, depending on the severity. After this time, you can reintroduce the eliminated foods one food, waiting two weeks in between each food to see if your symptoms return. If your symptoms return, then you should consider omitting that food from your diet entirely.

Let me be clear about what to expect in the upcoming thirty days—the first week is going to stink big time. You are not going to be happy with me, and you are probably going to have a tiny headache as your body adjusts to the diet changes. The second week will feel a little more comfortable, but you are still probably going to be slightly bitter about the entire process, and you are going to wonder why you started in the first place.

On day fifteen, you will get a burst of energy, and you will start to feel the effects of your hard work. You will feel like you are actually getting somewhere because you will be sleeping better and thinking clearer than you have in years. By the end of the fourth week, you are going to feel like a fabulous new person, and you are going to be jumping for joy!

Beyond Carrots Plan, Step 4: Planning for Success

After hearing that list of things that you should either discard or set to the side for the time being, you are probably wondering if there is anything left to eat. I have good news for you! The list of things that are approved on the *Beyond Carrots* Plan is extensive. I am going to list meats, fatty foods, fruit, starchy veggies, green leafy veggies, cancer-fighting cruciferous vegetables, *allum genus* plants (otherwise known as pee-you plants), and some other fun vegetables for you to explore in our journey together. I will give you a very brief description of how each of these foods benefits the eyes. Our goal here is to do what Hippocrates so eloquently stated, "Let food by thy medicine."

I found it particularly interesting that when I was forced to eliminate the chips and Diet Coke, I realized how many delicious fruits and veggies there are in the world. Discovering the beauty of these foods will take time, patience, and a shift in your thinking. As for recipes, quite frankly, I am not the best cook. When it comes to cooking and recipes, the internet is your friend! I have a ton of go-to YouTube channels and anti-inflammatory cooking blogs that I subscribe to get unique recipes. One such channel on YouTube that is fantastic for the amateur chef is Dani Spies's channel, Clean and Delicious.

So, let's dive into some of the foods that you can and should eat with the Beyond Carrots Plan:

Organic Meat

- **Grass-fed beef:** Grass-fed beef is an excellent source of protein. As it relates to eye health, beef is high in zinc which can help fight macular degeneration.
- **Grass-fed pork:** Grass-fed pork is high in vitamin B6 and B12, which are important for red blood cell production, and it helps keep your brain sharp. It is also high in zinc which can fight against macular degeneration.
- **Poultry:** Poultry such as chicken and turkey are also high in zinc,

helping defeat macular degeneration. So, next time you carve your Thanksgiving turkey, you know you are benefitting your eye health with your dinner.

- **Wild-caught fish (salmon, cod, trout, halibut, and sardines):** Wild-caught fish are high in omega-3 fatty acids, DHA, and EPA, which protect eyes against macular degeneration and reduce the risk of dry eye syndrome.

Fatty Foods That Don't Put on the Pounds

- **Avocado/Avocado oil:** Avocados are rich in antioxidants, lutein, and vitamin E. These antioxidants are some of the key players in conquering macular degeneration. Avocados also have a ton of vitamin K which can help reduce dark circles around the eyes. To get a quick fix of this vitamin, consider doing an avocado eye mask while you enjoy your margaritas and guacamole.
- **Coconut/coconut oil:** Coconuts are super fatty. But the fat in coconuts won't make you fat; rather, they will make you smart. Count me in on that one, right! The medium-chain triglycerides (MCTs) in coconuts have the potential to help prevent and reverse Alzheimer's and dementia.
- **Olive oil:** Olive oil reduces inflammation and helps reduce dry eye. Olive oil also helps to improve the body's absorption of lutein, a key nutrient that minimizes the risk of macular degeneration.
- **Olives:** Olives have a high content of vitamin A, a carotenoid that helps reduce the risk of developing macular degeneration.

Bring on the Colorful Veggies

- **Bok choy:** As far as eye health goes, bok choy is a superstar. With its high beta-carotene antioxidant levels and high levels of nutrients, it helps to protect the nerves and blood vessels in the back part of the eye. If that's not enough, bok choy is super high in the vital nutrients that promote healthy bone growth and glowing skin.
- **Broccoli/broccolini:** Remember the big "I" word that has been repeated like a broken record, *inflammation*? Well, broccoli and broccolini help to reduce inflammation while infusing the body with vital

nutrients and helping to fight cancer. Now that is a powerful vegetable.
- **Brussel sprouts:** This cancer-fighting superfood is jam-packed full of nutrients that help to reduce inflammation. Brussel sprouts are most notable for their high alpha-linolenic acid omega-3 fatty acid concentration. This plant-based version of the fatty acids often found in fish promotes brain, heart, and most importantly, eye health.
- **Cabbage:** Cabbage is super rich in our old favorite, beta-carotene. We know by now that beta-carotene aids in preventing macular degeneration and helps to delay the onset of cataracts.
- **Cauliflower:** Cauliflower is most notable for containing sulforaphane, a cancer-fighting chemical that gives cauliflower its distinct smell. Cauliflower also has a fair amount of fiber to help you poop. Who doesn't love that? Lastly, this superfood is chock-full of antioxidants to reduce inflammation and fight off disease.
- **Kale/spinach/collard greens:** Green leafy vegetables are high in carotenoids such as lutein and zeaxanthin, which protect the macula against macular degeneration. They also contain high amounts of vitamin A, further reducing the risk of macular degeneration and fighting against cataract formation.

Allum Genus Pee-You Plants

- **Garlic:** Garlic can help lower your blood pressure, and we know that high blood pressure is one of the Three Stooges that wreak havoc on the back part of the eyes. Furthermore, garlic can help reduce cholesterol, which is always a good thing when improving eye health.
- **Onions/shallots/leeks:** Onions and their cousins are another group of vegetables that do a number on your breath. Despite their off-putting smell, they are rich in cancer-fighting agents. The nutrients in onions and their cousins make them particularly good at lowering blood pressure. Furthermore, the green tops of onions are rich in beta-carotene, a quintessential nutrient for eye health.

Starchy Veggies—Who Needs Pasta?

- **Squash family:** There are two subsections of squash, summer squash and winter squash.
  - Summer squash family vegetables include zucchini and yellow squash. They are super good for the eyes. They are rich in vitamin C, folate, and beta-carotene. These are some of the key players in preserving eye health, especially vitamin C and beta-carotene.
  - Winter squash family vegetables include pumpkin, butternut squash, and spaghetti squash. Winter squash vegetables are also a great source of beta-carotene. Interesting to note that the more color the vegetable has, the more beta-carotene you will find. As a side note, be sure to bake or steam the winter squash family of vegetables as boiling them rids them of the nutrients. Also, the seeds in winter squash vegetables can be roasted, and they are a great source of minerals and protein.
- **Sweet Potatoes:** Talk about an eye health superfood! Sweet potatoes are one of the best foods that you can eat to promote healthy eyes. Just like we talked about in the winter squash vegetables, any time you see a vegetable that has a rich yellow color, you can guess that it is high in beta-carotene. We all know that beta-carotene is the preserver of our vision as it helps fight macular degeneration and delay cataract onset. Sweet potatoes also help to keep the gut nice and healthy. A healthy tummy leads to a healthy brain and healthy eyes. Boom! It does not get much better than that.

Other Fun Veggies

- **Artichokes:** Artichokes are one of the most antioxidant-rich vegetables on the farm stand. This is a nutrient-rich food that is fairly low calorie and relatively high protein as compared to other plant-based foods. Its high-fiber content keeps the tummy smiling. To top it all off, artichokes have been known to reduce blood pressure and lower cholesterol.
- **Asparagus:** Okay, Mom, listen up! Asparagus is a weight-loss food as it is low calorie and high in fiber! There is nothing Mom loves more than a weight-loss food. So, you can eat a ton of it and not exceed your calorie count for the day. It also helps to move things along the digestive tract, if you know what I mean. In doing so, it feeds the

good bacteria in the tummy, which helps keep the brain and eyes healthy. For pregnant women, asparagus is especially important as it is high in folate, which is necessary during the early stages of pregnancy to promote the baby's development.
- **Beets:** Beets are a pretty cool vegetable because they are jam-packed full of nutrients even though they are low in calories. Beets are some of the highest sugar content vegetables you can find. One fun experiment is watching your bowel and urine red when you eat a ton of beets. No, you are not bleeding. This is just the natural dye of the beets going in one end and coming out the other.
- **Carrots:** The mother of all eye health superfoods that needs no introduction, I present, CARROTS! Carrots have long been considered the one vegetable that helps preserve eye health. Carrots get their yellow-orange color from their crazy-high beta-carotene content. From macular degeneration to cataracts, pretty much every part of the eye benefits from this powerful nutrient. You could even go so far as to say that eating carrots can help to reduce your risk of developing night blindness. So, as grandma says, eat your carrots to keep your eyes healthy.

Fruit, Mother Earth's Dessert

- **Apple:** Have you ever noticed how well an apple curbs your appetite? Apples are great at making you feel full pretty quickly because they are high in fiber and fill that tummy to make you feel full. In addition, they are relatively nutritious, and the soluble fiber in apples helps to control cholesterol levels.
- **Bananas:** The most notable of the nutrients found in bananas is potassium. If you ever notice your eyelid twitching, you may have a slightly low potassium level, and the simple fix of eating a banana can, sometimes, help control the jiggly lids.
- **Berries (blackberries, blueberries, strawberries, raspberries):** Berries are another nutrient-rich fruit that is high in fiber and low in calories. You can tell by their dark color that they are rich in the good antioxidants that keep the eyes healthy. As a side note, the more color a food has, the better that food is for the eyes. If you diversify the color of foods you eat, you increase your chances of getting all of the

nutrients you need to have a balanced diet.
- **Citrus fruits (oranges, limes, lemons, tangerines, grapefruit):** You may have noticed a trend that foods yellow and orange are high in beta-carotene. Oranges are no exception. These antioxidants in citrus fruits help to reduce inflammation, and they work to reduce the risk of viral and bacterial infections.
- **Peaches:** Peaches are another fairly low-calorie source of antioxidants and fiber. They help nourish the gut and body and, most importantly, keep the eyes healthy.
- **Pears:** Pears are another great source of vitamins that are important to preserve eye health, such as vitamin A and vitamin C. Pears do a great job of feeding the good bacteria in the gut and softening the stool. The skin of pears is high in polyphenols, an antioxidant that helps to reduce inflammation and slow the aging process.

When You Need to Go

- **Apricots:** Apricots are high up there on the list of fruits that are good for the eyes. With the yellow color of an apricot, we know it is high in the antioxidants that keep the back part of the eye healthy: lutein and zeaxanthin. Since you can add in a little vitamin A and E to the mix with this fruit, you have a powerful, super delicious fruit. Apricots also have a fair amount of fiber, so don't eat too many unless you are mentally prepared to spend the afternoon on the toilet.
- **Cantaloupe:** There are few fruits that are better for the eyes than cantaloupe. Your grandma should be telling you to eat carrots with dinner and cantaloupe for dessert. Cantaloupe has more beta-carotene than most other fruits. It is also packed full of vitamin C, another big player when it comes to maintaining eye health.
- **Cherries:** Cherries are like dessert for the eyes. They are high in sugar, making them super sweet and delicious. At the same time, however, they are overflowing with our old friend, beta-carotene. You know the drill by now.
- **Figs:** Figs are my father's favorite! We oftentimes plan our trips to Italy around fig season. If you put my dad on the mountainside with a bunch of fig trees, he looks like a little kid in a candy store. Part of the reason why figs are so delicious is that they are very high in their

sugar content. Likewise, they are high in fiber.
- **Grapes:** Grapes are where it is at when looking to maintain eye health. If you were going to pick one fruit to consume daily to help reduce the risk of retina problems, grapes should be at the top of your list. They are high in bioflavonoids which are disease fighters. Bioflavonoids help reduce inflammation and prevent macular degeneration. Some people would prefer to eat their grapes, while others may prefer to drink them. Just remember to top it off at one serving. Cheers!
- **Honeydew:** Honeydew is a natural source of lutein and zeaxanthin, two very important antioxidants in maintaining eye health. You may recall us talking about these antioxidants in protecting our eyes against macular degeneration.
- **Kiwi:** Kiwi is another great source of vitamin C and fiber. This little fuzzball does a great job of protecting our eyeballs.
- **Mango:** Another great fruit for the eyes. Given their yellow color, I am sure you know what I am going to say. That's right! Mangos are rich in beta-carotene. Mangos are also high in fiber to help move things along the digestive tract.
- **Prunes:** Prunes are actually a hidden gem in the healthy eyes fruit list. Prunes are very high in beta-carotene, which is eventually converted to vitamin A. We know that beta-carotene is a macular degeneration fighting superhero.
- **Watermelon:** Watermelon has an antioxidant that we have not talked about too much, lycopene. This is the same antioxidant that you find in tomatoes. Lycopene helps fight diseases and maintain healthy eyes.

Spice It Up

- **Basil:** Basil has many antioxidants such as lutein and zeaxanthin that help protect the eye and reduce inflammation throughout the body.
- **Bay leaf:** Bay leaf is particularly good at helping to maintain blood sugar levels and control diabetes. It is also high in antioxidants.
- **Black pepper:** Black pepper is another spice that is particularly good at reducing inflammation because it is full of antioxidants.

- **Cilantro:** Cilantro has a fair amount of nutrients and does a great job of controlling inflammation.
- **Cinnamon:** If you were trying to decide which spice you should add to your daily life, look no further. Cinnamon is the big winner. Cinnamon has anti-inflammatory properties that trump many other spices. It is full of antioxidants that help to delay aging. Cinnamon helps control blood sugar and reduces the risk of heart disease.
- **Coriander:** Throwing a little coriander on your dish is a great way to help lower blood sugar levels and reduce inflammation. This will benefit your heart, brain, eyes, and body.
- **Cumin:** Cumin is an incredible spice as it has so many superpowers. Some people claim that cumin helps to reduce gastric upset and increase weight loss. Cumin can also moderate blood sugar levels. If that's not enough, cumin is rich in iron, so it helps in iron-deficient anemia.
- **Dill:** This delicious spice is especially useful in maintaining gut health and aiding in digestion. It will reduce gas and bloating and just make your tummy feel better. Dill is also a natural immune booster so consider adding it to your chicken soup when fighting a cold.
- **Ginger:** Ginger has grown quite the reputation for its ability to control nausea and reduce indigestion. It has been used to fight symptoms in illnesses from the common cold to bloating during menstruation. To top it all off, ginger is another powerful anti-inflammatory herb that adds a delicious touch to so many dishes.
- **Mint:** Mint is best known for its ability to reduce gastric upset. It is often added to tea when fighting nausea. Mint also has a fair amount of vitamin A, a key vitamin in preserving eye health.
- **Oregano:** Oregano is most acclaimed for its potential to fight bacterial infection. There certainly is some benefit to including oregano in your diet to get a few extra antioxidants and keep inflammation at bay.
- **Paprika:** Paprika is the mother of all spices when it comes to eye health as it is packed to the brim with lutein and zeaxanthin.
- **Parsley:** Parsley is one of those spices that is really good for eye health as it is high in lutein, zeaxanthin, and beta-carotene, three antioxidants that help protect our eyes against macular degeneration.

- **Saffron:** Saffron is one of those colorful spices that are high in the antioxidants that protect the eye called carotenoids. This spice helps reduce the aging process all over the body.
- **Sage:** Sage is an amazing herb with its ability to reduce inflammation. It has a significant amount of antioxidants to fight disease and delay the aging process.
- **Sea salt:** A little bit of salt is important in maintaining electrolyte balance. Try not to go overboard here, especially if you have a history of high blood pressure.
- **Thyme:** Thyme is an antioxidant-rich herb that also serves as an antifungal and antibacterial. Thyme is like a natural penicillin. As it relates to eye health, thyme is full of the nutrients that help protect our eyes.
- **Turmeric:** Turmeric is most popular for its ability to control inflammation. This powerful herb has been deemed helpful in minimizing damage in the eye ranging from retina problems to cataracts and dry eye.

Your Warm, Fuzzy Drinks

- **Bone broth:** Bone broth is fabulous for helping to repair the gut.
- **Chamomile tea:** Chamomile tea is best known for its calming properties that help promote a good night's sleep and soothe indigestion.
- **Decaf chai:** Believe it or not, you can find antioxidants that promote eye health in tea! Chai is a perfect example. This spicy, cozy drink is a great way to improve eye health in the form of a drink.
- **Green tea:** Green tea is the supreme anti-aging beverage. Its key ingredient is epigallocatechin-3-gallate (EGCG). This main component of green tea helps stop the damage done to your body with the aging process. This tea can be served warm or cold; either way, it will work its magic to help promote fat loss, increase metabolism, and improve memory function.

What to Do with the List above?

1. Eat a minimum of one serving of fish daily.

2. Eat one serving of meat daily (if you choose to be pescatarian, substitute this with fish).
3. Eat a healthy fat twice daily.
4. Eat as many green leafy vegetables as you can get your hands on, shooting for three handfuls per day.
5. Eat one or two servings of starchy veggies per day depending on your caloric needs.
6. Eat as many other vegetables as you can get your hands on, shooting for three servings per day.
7. Eat two to three servings of cancer-fighting foods daily.
8. Eat an *allum genus* (pee-you) plant once or twice daily.
9. Eat a ½ to one cup of fruit daily and try to limit fruit intake during the last two hours of your day.
10. Spice up as much as your heart desires while limiting salt intake when possible.
11. Consume two cups of bone broth daily. You may either make your own bone broth or buy high-quality powder bone broth. You may either drink this broth as a warming drink or add this broth to a recipe in place of water.
12. Drink a minimum of sixty-four ounces of water daily.

Have fun with your meal planning! There are so many amazing combinations of the spices and foods listed above it could make your head spin. You may need to think a little out of the box when it comes to breakfast. Traditional breakfast foods, including cereal, oatmeal, yogurt, and eggs, are not a good idea for the time you are following this protocol. You may find yourself eating some meat for breakfast with some greens in the form of a salad or a smoothie with some green leafy veggies, fruit, and flavorless bone broth powder. Filling each day with nutrient-rich food that heal our bodies from the inside out is the best way to feel energized and powerful.

Beyond Carrots Plan, Step 5: Get Out Those Tupperware Containers

The single best way to ensure that you stick to your plan is through meal prepping. If you do not have the meals at the tip of your fingers, I guarantee that your meal plan will go astray. A common misconception around meal prep is that you are obliged to eat the same thing every day when you prepare your food weekly. This is simply not true. You have endless flexibility around the foods you eat and the methods with which you prep your food. What is critical is that you have a plan and that you stick to it.

I grew up in an Italian house, and my mom spent three hours making dinner every night that always included a meat, vegetable, starch, and salad. I have been living on my own since I was eighteen, so I have learned to truly appreciate all the work she put into dinner each night. I have also concluded that I am simply never going to have three hours a night to cook dinner. Quite frankly, I barely have enough time to brown an onion when I get home from work at 7:00 p.m., and I have a two-year-old who wants to be held because he misses his mommy. I realize that the only way I am going to have my meals ready is by planning ahead. I will give you a wide range of ways to prep your meals, and you can decide what will work best for you.

Batch Prepping

One way to prepare your food for the week is by batch prepping different foods and creating combinations for different meals. For instance, you may decide to batch cooking chicken breast, roast vegetables, and prep fruit. You would then have these foods to use in your meals throughout the week. One potential drawback to this method of food prepping is that you will need to think a little bit harder each day about what is ready to eat and how to combine those foods. You will also have to go back to your checklist to ensure that you are getting the correct amounts of each type of food daily.

Container Prepping

If you are looking for a little more structure in your eating routine and do not mind some repetition in your meals as a trade for simplicity, container prepping may be right for you. In this method, you simply decide what you want to eat each meal and prepackage them in containers. You may even label these containers as breakfast, lunch, and dinner, so all you need to do is grab and go. Container prepping is as easy as fast food because it is literally ready to go in your refrigerator!

Mason Jar Salad Meals

A popular trend in container prepping is the mason jar salad. This has always been one of my favorites because it literally takes minutes to prep lunch for the week, and you can add versatility in the proteins and dressing. When I create my mason jar salads, I set up an assembly line with five jars, one for each day of the week. I stuff them full of all sorts of vegetables, occasionally adding fruit like diced apple or cranberries. I put the heavier foods on the bottom and layer up based on the weight of the vegetable. The top layer is always my green, leafy veggies. When I leave for work in the morning, all I need to do is grab a salad and a can of salmon or tuna, and I have my lunch. I have apple cider vinegar and oil at my office to use as a salad dressing. *Voila!* Lunch is served.

Freezer Meals

I recently discovered my new favorite dinner prep method, freezer meals. These meals are AMAZING! A freezer meal is a bunch of uncooked food tossed into a freezer bag and placed in the freezer. All you need to do in the morning is put the clump of food in the Crock-Pot or Instant Pot and roll. When you get home, you have a meal that tastes like you spent all day slaving in the kitchen. There are other freezer meals that you can let defrost in the refrigerator and grill or cook in the oven. Like I said, I like to do the bare minimum at night, so the Crock-Pot is my best friend.

You really cannot go wrong with any of these meal prep ideas as you have dinner at the tip of your fingers. However, the most important thing to remember when making your freezer meals is to label with explicit detail about what is in the freezer bag or container, cooking instructions, and expiration date. Although this may seem like a lot of work at the time, you will be happy when you know what you are cooking and how long it has been in the freezer.

Cook and Freeze

Unlike freezer meals where you literally put uncooked food in a bag and just freeze it, you have the option to cook and freeze your meals to eat on another night. Soups, stews, and sauces freeze very well and can be defrosted with ease. As with anything you put in the freezer, you must label these meals and give a "Use By" date, or they will be lost in the endless abyss of foods that you have stored in your freezer.

Meal Delivery Services

Perhaps the easiest way to ensure you have meals to eat every day is to get a meal delivery service. Because I am single, and it feels like cooking for one at the end of a long day seems like way too much work, I have toyed around with various meal delivery services over the years. I can tell you that these services have come a long way from where they were a decade ago. With many services, you have the option to request various food preferences from gluten-free and dairy-free to vegan and pescatarian. You may even have the option to omit various foods from your diet. Most delivery companies tell you the macronutrient and dietary information for each meal. They adjust the serving size to meet your caloric intake goals.

One of the drawbacks to meal delivery services is, obviously, the cost. It is not cheap to have someone grocery shop, cook, and set your meals on your doorstep. However, it is not a bad option for those who have very limited to shop and cook.

The method that you use to prep your meals is unimportant. You may even decide on a combination of various prep methods. What matters most is that you create a plan and stick to it! Your success with the *Beyond Carrots* Plan depends on you deciding what you will do and making it happen.

Beyond Carrots Plan, Step 6: KISS Vitamins

I have always said that the majority of the vitamins and nutrients that we give our bodies should be from the food we eat. Even with the best diet ever, there are four essential supplements in the *Beyond Carrots* Plan that are necessary to aid in the healing process. We are going to KISS (Keep It Simple, Silly), so you do not need to break the bank and take a million pills. Each of these supplements is hand-picked to help reverse diseases and help you regain vitality. Before you begin any supplementation plan, you should discuss the regimen with your primary care physician.

Fish Oil

Fish oil is the mother of all inflammatory reducing supplements and a quintessential supplement in the *Beyond Carrots* Plan. It aids in reducing disease from your heart to your brain and everywhere in between. If that's not enough, fish oil helps to heal your gut and lubricate your joints. Some of the many eye conditions that are positively impacted by taking fish oil are dry eye disease, macular degeneration, blood clots in the eye, and blood vessel damage due to hypertension.

If you ever look closely at the fish oil container, you may notice that the oil is described as containing EPA (eicosapentaenoic acid) and DHA (docosahexaenoic acid). You want to take a minute to look closely at the actual amount of EPA/DHA in the fish oil you are taking because 1,000 mg of fish oil does not always mean that you are getting 1,000 mg of the active ingredients, EPA/DHA. In the *Beyond Carrots* Plan, 2,000–4,000 mg of combined EPA/DHA are to be taken daily.

One common concern I hear when I discuss fish oil supplementation with my patients is foul fish taste and burping fish oil that some people experience. If you freeze your fish oil, you will practically eliminate the burping because it takes a minute for the fish oil to defrost in your tummy. Also, if you eat a little something before and after your fish oil pills, you create a cushion for oil in your stomach and do not taste it as much.

Probiotics

When it comes to healing your gut, I cannot repeat myself enough. The gut is where inflammation begins, and we must heal the gut if we want to heal the eyes. If you recall our chapter on gut health, the stomach is packed with good bacteria that help to protect our bodies. The goal of probiotics is to increase the size of this good bacteria army.

The good bacteria in the gut are destroyed so easily by many factors, from oral antibiotics to elevated stress levels. Even if you think you have the healthiest stomach in the world, it is recommended that you take probiotics daily. The quality of the probiotics is graded by the number of CFU of various bacteria. When you go shopping for probiotics, make sure that there is a minimum of 50 billion CFU per capsule. In the *Beyond Carrots* Plan, it is recommended that you take one probiotic morning and night. Try to take your probiotics at the same time each day because your body needs that constant support from the outside troops.

Vitamin D

Vitamin D is one of the most important vitamins you can take because low vitamin D levels are linked to countless medical conditions. Osteoporosis, diabetes, dementia, heart disease, depression, and even cancer are linked to low vitamin D levels. Vitamin D affects every system of our bodies, and the eyes are no exception. Dry eye, macular degeneration, and diabetic eye disease are just a few eye diseases that have links to inflammation and may be impacted by vitamin D levels.

As part of your baseline testing, you will be getting your vitamin D levels assessed with your bloodwork analysis. If you are an exception to the norm and have acceptable vitamin D levels in your bloodwork, there is no need to supplement. Most people will find that their vitamin D levels are low, and supplementation is indicated. The *Beyond Carrots* Plan calls for 1,000 IU of vitamin D daily. You should take vitamin D alongside a meal with some healthy fats to make sure that you get the biggest bang for your buck because vitamin D is absorbed into your body best when it is around fats.

Eye Vitamins

At the heart of reversing eye disease is a group of antioxidants whose main function is to protect the back part of the eye. These antioxidants can reverse damage to the eye and help to repair the nerves of the retina. Research has shown that supplementation with eye vitamins can improve vision even when the eye is perfectly healthy from the start.

The antioxidants that directly affect the eyes are carotenoids, and they include lutein, zeaxanthin, meso-zeaxanthin, and astaxanthin. Some of the most powerful combinations of these antioxidants are only available through your eye doctor. If you cannot receive a prescription-strength eye vitamin, there are many great options over the counter. The most referenced study when creating eye vitamins is the AREDS 2 study, so long as the vitamins you chose are in coherence with this study, you will protect your eyes. Like vitamin D, eye vitamins should be taken with your meal with some healthy fats because they are absorbed by your body best when surrounded by fat.

So, to review, the four supplements that recommended in the *Beyond Carrots* Plan are fish oil (2,000–4,000 mg), probiotics (50 billion CFU), vitamin D (1,000 IU), and eye vitamins. All of these supplements should be taken with food to maximize absorption. The only supplement that must be taken twice daily is the probiotics. The goal here is to take as few supplements as possible to restore our bodies, brains, and eyes without breaking the bank.

Beyond Carrots Plan, Step 7: Get Off Your Butt

When you think about going to the gym, you probably think about building your arms and legs or flattening your abs. You may crave that runner's high you get at the end of your jog. The last thing you probably think about when you hit the weights is your eyes. I am here to tell you that every square inch of your body is affected by your workouts.

First and foremost, exercise reduces levels of the stress hormone cortisol. Maintaining a healthy cortisol level helps reduce inflammation, improve sleep, control depression, and increase weight loss. Each of these factors either directly or indirectly impact eye health. When cortisol levels creep up, you are like a walking time bomb just waiting for inflammation and disease to occur in any area of your body. I can assure you, by following the guidelines in the *Beyond Carrots* Plan, you will tame the cortisol monster in your body, and you will feel like a new person!

Cardiovascular activity also brings new blood to every organ in your body, including your eyes. The improved blood flow can help to improve vision and reduce the risk of developing glaucoma. Studies have shown that exercise can reduce the pressure in the eyes in patients who have glaucoma! Can you imagine being able to throw away your glaucoma medications just because you get regular cardiovascular exercise?

Studies also show that regular exercise can go so far as to prevent the onset of type 2 diabetes. With exercise, we can better control blood sugar and reduce the unneeded fat around our bodies, which can help manage diabetes. We all know by now the devastating effect that diabetes can have on the back part of the eye. Regardless of whether or not you have received an official diagnosis of being diabetic, regular exercise is critical to maintaining control of your blood sugar levels and reducing your chances of losing your sight.

If that's not enough to get you off your butt, studies show that you have a reduced risk of developing macular degeneration if you get regular physical activity. There was a huge study done in Beaver Dam, Wisconsin, with 3,874 people between the ages of forty-three and eighty-six. These people were evaluated every five years for fifteen years. The scientists were astonished when they discovered that the incidence of a type of macular degeneration was reduced by thirty percent over fifteen years for those individuals who walked more than twelve blocks daily.

The science behind the magic of exercise as it relates to macular degeneration is not fully established. It could be the increased blood flow to the eye, the reduced inflammation, or just better cardiovascular health. Even though we are still working out the biology behind the results, the studies are clear—get moving to reduce your risk of blindness due to macular degeneration.

I am not going to refer to this step in the *Beyond Carrots* Plan by the big "E" because it has such a bad connotation. I mean, who wants to exercise? Exercise is work, and work is no fun. We are going to get out and enjoy the world by getting off our butts and moving more. This subtle shift in perspective around what you are doing when you move your body creates a more positive vibe around the idea of exercising.

If you were to go to the American Heart Association and ask them how much you should work out per week, they would give you specific guidelines. They would tell you that you should be getting a hundred and fifty minutes of moderate aerobic exercise per week or seventy-five minutes of vigorous aerobic exercise per week. They would also mention that you should squeeze in moderate to high-intensity strength training two days per week. Many people are already meeting these criteria in their workout regimen. If that is you, then you get a big high-five. Most people are not meeting these workout criteria.

To the overweight individual who has not worked out in years and can barely walk around the block, the thought of moderate aerobic exercise is paralyzing. To the marathon runner or Olympic swimmer, these criteria are surpassed daily and with ease. We are all starting from a different place, so the *Beyond Carrots* Plan recommends that you just move your body for thirty minutes per day. If you enjoy being outside, go for a brisk walk for thirty minutes per day. You can mix it up and consider a nature walk or a walk on the beach if you have those options available. If you enjoy shopping as much as my mom, walking around a mall will make the time will fly! For me, swimming and yoga are like pure bliss. It does not matter what you do during these thirty minutes of your day. What matters most is that you find something to do that gets you moving and makes you happy.

As part of the *Beyond Carrots* Plan, we are going to monitor your heart rate as you are moving. We want to monitor the heart rate because we want to see what effect our movement has on our bodies. When you see your heart rate go up, your heart is saying, "Thank you so much for remembering that I am alive!" There is a party inside your body every time your heart rate goes up a little bit, and your body is having an absolute blast! To know that your body is having the best rage ever, subtract your age from 220 and divide by two. This is the minimum number we are shooting for as we move on a daily basis. You will find the more parties you have in your body, the longer it takes your heart rate to hit that magic number.

When it comes to getting your body moving during your *Beyond Carrots* journey, more and harder is not always better. Especially during this time that you are trying to heal the body, it is important that you keep your movement low-impact and moderate-intensity. Now is not the time to set out to run a marathon or try to keep up with the heavyweights at the gym. I will tell you a secret. I found out that I had my potentially blinding eye disease approximately six months after I joined an extremely high-intensity workout gym that was very popular across America at the time. I believe that my untrained body could not handle the physical exertion during these extreme workouts. It is likely that the stress I was putting on my body coupled with some mild inflammation resulted in a breakdown in the blood vessels in my eyes. Don't make the same mistake. Know your limits and keep things moderate.

Make sure to plan the workout into your day. If you do not plan this part of your day and build it into your routine, there is a good chance that the million and one things that you need to do will get in the way of your "you time." The more you make your movement time a habit, the more ingrained your workout will become into your day. I know it sounds easier said than done, but I promise you will begin to love this time, especially if you design it around something you enjoy, such as being outside, watching TV, or swimming.

Beyond Carrots Plan, Step 8: Take 10

You already understand the importance of meditation and prayer, especially as it relates to eye health. Taking this step of the *Beyond Carrots* Plan seriously will reduce your risk of a potentially blinding cardiovascular disease, manage diabetes, lower inflammation, decrease dry eye, and reduce the risk of macular degeneration. Not only that, but meditation is also free and convenient. You do not need to buy any fancy equipment. All you need to do is take ten minutes to yourself daily.

The first step to meditation is picking a time, place, and form of meditation and planning it into your day. You should also come up with a backup plan, just in case your first plan flops for one reason or another. Shoot to make a period of mindfulness part of your morning routine. If you can also work it into your bedtime ritual, that would be awesome, but the morning routine sets the mindset for your entire day.

How long you spend in meditation is completely up to you. I know that when I started meditating, I could barely sit for ten minutes. Quite frankly, I still cannot sit for over ten minutes on some days. In my practice, every day is slightly different in the length of time that I spend meditating. What I have kept consistent in my practice is the time of the day that I spend in solitude.

Beyond Carrots Plan, Step 9: Assess Your Progress

Now comes the fun part when we get to see how well we did and reap the rewards of the hard work! Every thirty days, you will assess your progress to see how your body is responding to the *Beyond Carrots* Plan. I am using thirty days as our marker because there is a lot of change that can happen in your body in just thirty days. It is important that you stay on track in your journey and resist the urge to jump the gun in evaluating your progress before the 30-day mark. You will need every single one of your thirty days to get measurable results.

At the end of the time allotted, request that your eye doctor and medical doctor repeat all baseline tests performed at the beginning of the *Beyond Carrots* Plan.

Eye Doctor

1. Visual acuity with and without glasses
2. Glasses prescription
3. Schirmer's test
4. Eye Health Evaluation: Slit Lamp Exam and Retina Evaluation
5. Ocular Coherence Tomography (OCT) (if available)
6. Contrast sensitivity and MPOD (if available)

Medical Doctor

1. Inflammatory markers: CRP and ESR
2. Blood sugar levels: Hba1C and fasting blood sugar level
3. Cholesterol
4. Blood pressure
5. Vitamin D, specifically 1.25-dihydroxy vitamin D
6. Fish oil: EPA and DHA in the blood

You will also be repeating all of the tests that you did at home:

1. Measure your body weight
2. BMI
3. Measure your waist circumference
4. Measure bowel transit time after eating one cup of beets
5. Complete the Perceived Stress Scale Test
6. Complete the *Beyond Carrots* Inflammatory Questionnaire

CONGRATULATIONS! You have completed the first phase of the *Beyond Carrots* journey!

Our goal is to see that at the end of the thirty days, you will have one or more items that improved from your baseline. Any movement towards a healthier body and mind is a movement towards healthier eyes. Although everyone should see improvement in one or more areas of the baseline tests, not everyone will be able to reverse eye disease completely in just thirty days, but you always have another thirty days to improve your eyes and body further. The fact that you can look at these baseline tests and see some movement to a healthier body is enough to keep us motivated to repeat our efforts and continue to reverse eye disease.

Beyond Carrots Plan, Step 10: Reward Yourself!

Here comes the best part of the plan that absolutely must not be skipped! Every week that you have successfully completed the *Beyond Carrots* Plan, you get to reward yourself. I can tell you, firsthand, that sticking to the program takes a solid vision, planning, and discipline. The best way to ensure that you continue to stay on track is to be sure that you recognize and congratulate yourself. It is this positive reinforcement that will drive you for the entire thirty days.

It would help if you chose a reward that is healthy and revitalizing. There are so many ways to congratulate yourself that do not involve junk food, alcohol, or other unhealthy habits. The goal here is to give yourself life and happiness because you just did something remarkable for your body. I can assure you, eating a dozen donuts or drinking a bottle of wine will not bring your life and happiness. You will feel disgusting, and you will wonder what the heck you were thinking.

Some healthy rewards for you to consider are the following:
1. Go shopping!
2. Build a Zen area in your home with candles, a waterfall, and a yoga mat.
3. Treat yourself to an at-home spa day with a bubble bath.
4. Take a day off and go for a walk on the beach or in a nature preserve.
5. Get a massage.
6. Watch a funny movie. Laughter truly is the best medicine.
7. Make yourself a surf and turf dinner with lobster and filet mignon.
8. Go for a day trip to a nearby town where you can escape your day-to-day routine.
9. See your favorite band at an outdoor live show.
10. Enjoy a game night with your family and friends.
11. Read a book and listen to classical music.
12. Go camping! The great outdoors brings life!

13. Take your dream vacation.
14. Invest in a piece of workout gear.
15. Just do nothing. You deserve this time to yourself.

You know you better than I know you. Pick a reward that will have you smiling for days so that you will eventually come to associate your hard work with the ultimate reward that is to come. You got this! Stick with it!

Baby Steps *Beyond Carrots* Plan

Now let me tell you about a modified version of that plan that may be more suitable for the individual who is not prepared to go gung-ho with the complete *Beyond Carrots* Plan. This is still going to be work, so don't think you are getting off light. To reiterate, this is meant to be a lifelong change to your eating patterns and lifestyle choices that is sustainable. Many small changes made over the course of the year will result in massive changes in your mind and body. Trust me! I know you should never trust someone who says, "trust me," but that does not count in this situation.

Step 1: Find Your "Why" and Define Your Goals

Before you do anything at all, you have to make your mind up that you want to change. If you are teeter-tottering and not fully committed to adjusting your diet and reducing your chances of eye disease and other medical problems, you will cave at the first temptation. Consider your motivating factors and your goals and jot them down somewhere. By motivating factors, I mean, get to the heart of the WHY that drives you to make a change. As for your goals, be as specific as possible. Some people like using yellow pads; others use the notes app in their phones. I do not care where you write it down; just get your words physically written somewhere. You are far more likely to succeed if you do not skip this step.

Step 2: Baseline Testing

I am going to keep this super simple. The only two stops you need to make are to your local optometrist and to your primary care doctor. If you have not already gotten your annual eye exam and yearly physical, there is no better time than now. You may want to do some quick research on your eye doctor to ensure that they have the most advanced technology that will simplify your eye exam experience with equipment such as a wide field retina camera.

Aside from the doctor visits, there are three things at home that you should do that will take no more than five minutes.

1. Weigh yourself
2. Take a picture of your face and body
3. Measure your waist circumference, the distance around your waist right at your belly button.

Just so you know, I am giving you this homework because I project that you will see some improvement in one or all of these categories as you work your way through the Baby Steps *Beyond Carrots* Plan. It is quite likely that you will see some weight reduction as you begin to make healthier food choices. Your complexion and body appearance will also probably improve because you will be consuming foods that energize and revitalize. Lastly, I predict that the distance around your waist will decrease. Believe it or not, waist circumference is a key indicator of morbidity or how long you will live. So, needless to say, this number is pretty important.

See, this plan is not too difficult. You can probably get all of that done in a matter of no time and with little effort. So now, let's get down to the nitty-gritty.

Step 3: Spring Cleaning

I have given you a detailed list of foods to avoid at all costs. It is, I admit, overwhelming. I needed to list all of those toxic foods because if you are on the road to blindness, you have to put the brakes on and stop the destruction of the body. However, not everyone is on that path.

In the Baby Steps Plan, you will pick out one or two toxic foods that you see yourself eating and eliminate them from your diet. For the first month, I would advise that you choose an easy food to eliminate. Chose a food that you eat maybe once a week and would not be a huge adjustment if you were to cut that food or beverage out of your system entirely. Remember, the name of the game here is Baby Steps. You may choose to cut out chips or cookies, soft drinks, pastries, or even just cut one soft drink out of your day if you are a heavy soda drinker. Every baby step counts!

You are probably wondering where I am going with this plan, as you cannot reverse eye disease by cutting out one soda from your diet. Hang in there; you will see the big picture in a little bit.

Step 4: Add Nutritious Foods

This step is kind of fun. You get to look through the list of foods that are good for you and pick out one or two foods that you are not eating or eating very little of and add them to your diet. I know this does not sound too exciting, but it can be super fun to check out different foods. For instance, I randomly picked up a spaghetti squash when trying to reverse my own eye disease. I had to Google how to even cook it. It turns out spaghetti squash is delicious; who knew?

This step aims to add healthy foods to your everyday diet that will, eventually, serve to replace the unhealthy foods. I am requesting that you work with only one or two foods for now. We want to make these goals achievable because when you finish a month of change and pat yourself on the back, you will feel motivated to proceed with your next baby step in the plan.

Step 5: Get Out Those Tupperware Containers

The best way to ensure success with the Baby Steps *Beyond Carrots* Plan is to plan ahead. If you do not remove the bad foods from your line of sight and do not make your healthy foods easily accessible, you are likely to fail miserably. Likewise, planning ahead is an absolute must. Now, some people have all day to go grocery shopping and cook. I, on the other hand, am a very busy person. I barely have time to make it to the grocery store once a week. When you add food prep and clean up, it becomes a hopeless cause to achieve on a daily basis. A general rule of thumb is to make sure that by 11 a.m. every day, you know what you are having for dinner, and you have a plan to easily put that dinner together when it is time to eat.

Step 6: KISS Vitamins

In the KISS vitamin section, we outlined four vitamins that are important to maintaining the healthiest eyes possible. Those vitamins were fish oil, vitamin D, probiotics, and eye vitamins. As much as I would like to simplify this step further, I just cannot. It is just as easy to pop four vitamins as it is to pop one. The challenge in taking vitamins is building the habit of taking the vitamins into your routine in the morning. If you are going to get into the habit of taking vitamins, you are best off just getting used to taking all of them at the same time.

Step 7: Get Off Your Butt

The key here is to make movement every day a part of your routine. As part of the Baby Steps *Beyond Carrots* Plan, make sure that you set a minimum of ten to fifteen minutes aside daily to do some physical activity. Try to keep a consistent time for your workout so that it becomes part of your daily habit. I know that your doctor will tell you that thirty minutes a day of moderate-intensity exercise is critical to maintaining heart and bone health. I just think that thirty minutes can be daunting to some people.

There are two reasons why I suggest ten to fifteen minutes of movement in the Baby Step Plan. First of all, when you set out to do ten to fifteen minutes of working out, you will probably find that, before you know it, it has been thirty to forty-five minutes. Secondly, I think that the biggest challenge that most people have when working out is building it into their daily routine. When it is as ritualized as brushing your teeth in the morning, you are much more likely to fulfill your workout plan. For that reason, I recommend starting off with ten to fifteen minutes every day to have solid practice. From there, you can add time and intensity.

Step 8: Take 10

Ten minutes of "me time" sounds like a dream to some people. It may sound next to impossible to add a chunk of time to just chill to your day. I totally get it. Again, the main goal in the Baby Step Plan is to build habits that last. For that reason, I would recommend that you start off by taking only five minutes to just chill, by yourself, in quiet solitude and just relax. In this time, you can pray, journal, sit in complete silence, listen to relaxing music, do restorative yoga poses, take a stroll, or do whatever calms your mind. If you do this daily, I 100% guarantee that your stress levels will decrease, and you will begin to cherish this precious time. Before you know it, you will find yourself extending this treasured chance to relax to ten minutes or longer.

Step 9: Assess Progress

The first day of each month is your day to assess progress. This is a time to check in with yourself and see how you feel. Do you notice any changes in your complexion, body, bowel movements, mood, or overall cravings with the changes made over the past month? I am always a big fan of writing things down so that you can use this information as a reference point for months to come.

Hop on the scale and see what the scale says. Remember, this is just a number and not always indicative of the level of progress made during the month. Repeat your photos of your body and face so that you can see a side-by-side comparison of what you looked like a month ago.

As for doctors' appointments, in the Baby Steps *Beyond Carrots* Plan, it is recommended that you repeat your physical and eye exam every six months. It is a good idea to go back sooner than a year because if you are following the plan carefully, you may see changes in bloodwork numbers and eye exam results in this short period of time. These changes will motivate you to keep charging forward.

After you have spent some time assessing progress, take a moment to consider what areas of the plan are working for you and how you can push yourself just a little bit to grow on the previous months' accomplishments. Consider each of the following:

- What toxic foods can you add to the list of foods that you have eliminated from your diet?
- What nutritious foods can you add to your daily regimen?
- What meals can you plan ahead of time to eliminate the chances of making bad food choices?
- Can you add five minutes of moderate-intensity exercise to your workout routine?
- Can you add two minutes of solitude to your relation time?

By taking a moment to answer each of these five questions monthly, you will build habits and notice compounding changes over the course of a year. This will result in habits that last a lifetime and continual growth. Furthermore, when you see yourself set out to make subtle modifications and succeed, you will have a feeling of accomplishment, and this will fuel your transformation.

Step 10: Reward Yourself!

Do not forget the most important step of all! Reward yourself for any small step that you made towards a healthier you. Even if you set out to make a change in your diet and you slipped up once or twice, you still made progress. Change does not happen overnight, so do not beat yourself up over a lapse or two. Becoming more aware of the foods that you are putting into your body is a baby step towards the disease-free, energetic, happy version of you that will come with the dedication and hard work in the Baby Steps *Beyond Carrots* Plan.

Conclusion: I Am SOOOOO Grateful

Several years ago, a dear friend gave me a silver paperweight that reads "SOOOOOO GRATEFUL." This gentle reminder makes me think about all the amazing people in my life who have been a part of my journey. I could not be luckier to be surrounded by people who truly care about me and are there for me through my life's challenges.

First and foremost, I want to thank my one and only two-year-old son, Zachary Joseph Caruso, for sharing his mommy time so that the vision and lives of people all over the world can be helped. Zachary has brought me the gift of endless love in the form of big hugs and belly laughs. Being a single mom by choice has required me to be more disciplined than I have ever been in the past. Interestingly, this structure has forced me to be more diligent about my yoga and meditation practice to instill a sense of calm in my every action.

Thank you, also, to my mom, who has always encouraged me to be the best doctor, mother, and person that I can possibly be. I am sure watching me go through my challenges with my eyes was more difficult for my mother than it was for me. Yet, she remained strong and had full faith in my ability to overcome my obstacles. Without her support, I would not be where I am today. Mom spent countless hours changing diapers and entertaining my munchkin while I typed away in my office.

My father is the hardest working individual that I know. He came to America from Italy when he was ten years old and became very successful through his hard work, dedication, and perseverance. I emulate his every action in my work ethic, and I would not be up at 5:00 a.m. writing a book if not for my father as a role model.

My family has always been incredibly important to me. I could not be more grateful for the support and love that I receive from my brother, Tony, his wife, Megan, and their little boys, Sebastian and Miles.

From the bottom of my heart, I would like to thank all of the doctors at Bascom Palmer Eye Institute of Palm Beach Gardens, Florida. Every single individual at Bascom Palmer Eye Institute naturally maintains a special personal touch with each patient who walks through their door. The level of patient care is consistent from the clinical administrator, Jennifer McGee, to the ophthalmologists and technicians. like Dr. Thomas Albini in retina and Dr. David Greenfield in glaucoma. It is incredible for a large ophthalmology clinic to maintain this level of rapport with its patients. I can tell you from my experiences, the emotion that goes into potential vision loss is extreme. The amount of time that the institute took to comfort me with warm hugs and caring touches will never be forgotten.

When I graduated from optometry school seventeen years ago, my main goal was to bring happiness to as many people as possible by giving better sight. I cannot thank Target Optical and Luxottica Eye Care enough for providing me a means of making this dream come true at my practice, Caruso Eye Care. Target Optical has supported the development of my practice and has provided me with the resources to grow and impact the lives of thousands. Through OneSight, a Luxottica Eye Care affiliate program, I was even able to travel to Tanzania and give free eye exams and glasses to over 3,500 in five days. I could not be more blessed for all of the relationships that I have built with wonderful people at Target Optical throughout the years.

I would also like to recognize all of my educators throughout the years. Their hard work and dedication have shaped me as a physician. Through the American Academy of Anti-Aging and Regenerative Medicine, I learned about nutrition and its impact on our health. That served as the framework for much of the information in this book.

I believe that my quest for knowledge began at the Illinois College of Optometry (ICO), where I had teachers who truly cared about me as an individual. In the words of my dear friend and professor at ICO, Dr. David Lee, "I want you to always be in search for the truth. In all of your research and in everything you do, continue to question until you find the truth." He told me that role of the professors at ICO was to provide scientific foundation. It was up to me to question those theories and expand my knowledge base every single day of my optometric career.

I would also like to thank my publishing company, Mindstir Media, for putting the best team together to bring my book to life and having faith that it will make it into the hands of many. Your systematic approach to publication puts me at ease and your marketing team truly "gets it." My book would be sitting on the desktop of my computer collecting dust if not for the expertise of your professionals.

I want to thank God for being there as my companion through every minute of every day of my life. Although we all may not believe in God as our higher power, it has become so clear to me that everything happens for a reason. It was not by chance that the one body part affected by my inflammation was in my area of expertise. I believe that my higher power saw the eye disease coming my way and picked me to be the bearer of this affliction because it would make me grow stronger.

What seemed like the worst day of my life was actually a miracle in a way that I would only fully understand upon the completion of my book. The true miracle will come to fruition when I see the impact that my work has on its readers. So thank you, too.

Bibliography

Abdel-Aal, e., Akhtar, H., Zaheer, K., & Ali, R. (2013). Dietary sources of lutein and zeaxanthin carotenoids and their role in eye health. *Nutrients*, 5(4), 1169–1185. https://doi.org/10.3390/nu5041169.

Achamrah, N., Déchelotte, P., & Coëffier, M. (2017). Glutamine and the regulation of intestinal permeability: from bench to bedside. *Current opinion in clinical nutrition and metabolic care*, 20(1), 86–91. https://doi.org/10.1097/MCO.0000000000000339.

Acheson, K.J., Gremaud, G., Meirim, I., et al. (2004). Metabolic effects of caffeine in humans: lipid oxidation or futile cycling? *The American journal of clinical nutrition*, 79(1), 40–46. https://doi.org/10.1093/ajcn/79.1.40.

Aeberli, I., Gerber, P.A., Hochuli, M., Kohler, S., et al. (2011). Low to moderate sugar-sweetened beverage consumption impairs glucose and lipid metabolism and promotes inflammation in healthy young men: a randomized controlled trial. *The American journal of clinical nutrition*, 94(2), 479–485. https://doi.org/10.3945/ajcn.111.013540.

Age-Related Eye Disease Study Research Group. (2001). A Randomized, Placebo-Controlled, Clinical Trial of High-Dose Supplementation With Vitamins C and E, Beta Carotene, and Zinc for Age-Related Macular Degeneration and Vision Loss: AREDS Report No. 8. *Arch Ophthalmologica*, 119(10), 1417–1436. doi:10.1001/archopht.119.10.1417.

Age-Related Eye Disease Study 2 (AREDS2) Research Group. (2014). Secondary analyses of the effects of lutein/zeaxanthin on age-related macular degeneration progression: AREDS2 report No. 3. *JAMA Ophthalmology*, 132(2), 142–149. https://doi.org/10.1001/jamaophthalmol.2013.7376.

Amagase, H., Petesch, B. L., Matsuura, H., Kasuga, S., & Itakura, Y.

(2001). Intake of garlic and its bioactive components. *The Journal of nutrition, 131*(3s), 955S–62S. https://doi.org/10.1093/jn/131.3.955S.

American Chemical Society Meeting & Exposition, Washington, D.C., Aug. 27-Sept. 1, 2005. News release, American Chemical Society.

American Heart Association, https://www.ahajournals.org/doi/abs/10.1161/circulationaha.107.185649

Appleby, P.N., Allen, N.E., Key, T.J. (2011). Diet, vegetarianism, and cataract risk. *The American Journal of Clinical Nutrition, 93*(5), 1128-1135. https://doi.org/10.3945/ajcn.110.004028.

Ashraf, R., Khan, R. A., Ashraf, I., & Qureshi, A. A. (2013). Effects of Allium sativum (garlic) on systolic and diastolic blood pressure in patients with essential hypertension. *Pakistan journal of pharmaceutical sciences, 26*(5), 859–863.

Assini, J.M., Mulvihill, E.E., & Huff, M.W. (2013). Citrus flavonoids and lipid metabolism. *Current opinion in lipidology, 24*(1), 34–40. https://doi.org/10.1097/MOL.0b013e32835c07fd.

Ayaki, M., Tsubota, K., Kawashima, M., et al. (2018). Sleep Disorders are a Prevalent and Serious Comorbidity in Dry Eye. *Investigative Ophthalmology and Visual Science, 59*(14), DES143-DES150. https://doi.org/10.1167/iovs.17-23467.

Bagheri, N., Wajda, B., Calvo, C., & Durrani, A. (Eds.). (1998). *The Wills Eye Manual: Office and emergency room diagnosis and treatment of eye disease* (pp. 393-432). Lippincott Williams and Wilkins.

Bahn R.S. (2010). Graves' ophthalmopathy. *The New England journal of medicine, 362*(8), 726–738. https://doi.org/10.1056/NEJMra0905750.

Bajgai, P., Katoch, D., Dogra, M.R., & Singh, R. (2017). Idiopathic retinal vasculitis, aneurysms, and neuroretinitis (IRVAN) syndrome: clinical perspectives. *Clinical ophthalmology (Auckland, N.Z.), 11*, 1805–1817. https://doi.org/10.2147/OPTH.S128506.

Balakireva, A.V., & Zamyatnin, A.A. (2016). Properties of Gluten Intolerance: Gluten Structure, Evolution, Pathogenicity and Detoxification Capabilities. *Nutrients, 8*(10), 644. https://doi.org/10.3390/nu8100644.

Basu, A., Devaraj, S., & Jialal, I. (2006). Dietary factors that promote or retard inflammation. *Arteriosclerosis, thrombosis, and vascular biology, 26*(5), 995–1001. https://doi.org/10.1161/01.ATV.0000214295.86079.d1.

Belizário, J.E., & Faintuch, J. (2018). Microbiome and Gut Dysbiosis. *Experientia supplementum (2012), 109*, 459–476. https://doi.org/10.1007/978-3-319-74932-7_13.

Berger, J., Shepard, D., Morrow, F., et al. (1989). Relationship between dietary intake and tissue levels of reduced and total vitamin C in the nonscorbutic guinea pig. *Journal of Nutrition, 119*(5), 734–740.

Bologna, E. Use and Abuse of Alcohol in Italy. *Instituto Nazionale di Statistica*. April 16, 2015. Retrieved from https://www.istat.it/en/archive/156232.

Borek C. (2006). Garlic reduces dementia and heart-disease risk. *The Journal of nutrition, 136*(3 Suppl), 810S–812S. https://doi.org/10.1093/jn/136.3.810S.

Brice, C.F., Smith, A.P. (2002). Effects of caffeine on mood and performance: a study of realistic consumption. *Psychopharmacology, 164*, 188–192. https://doi.org/10.1007/s00213-002-1175-2.

Carding, S., Verbeke, K., Vipond, D.T., Corfe, B.M., & Owen, L.J. (2015). Dysbiosis of the gut microbiota in disease. *Microbial ecology in health and disease, 26*, 26191. https://doi.org/10.3402/mehd.v26.26191.

Chiu, C.J., Taylor, A. (2007). Nutritional Antioxidants and Age-related Cataract and Maculopathy. *Experimental Eye Research, 84*(2), 229-245. https://

doi.org/10.1016/j.exer.2006.05.015.

Cos, P., De Bruyne, T., Hermans, N., Apers, S., Berghe, D. V., & Vlietinck, A. J. (2004). Proanthocyanidins in health care: current and new trends. *Current medicinal chemistry*, *11*(10), 1345–1359. https://doi.org/10.2174/0929867043365288.

Cumming, R.G., Mitchell, P., Smith, W. (2000). Diet and Cataract: The Blue Mountains Eye Study. *Ophthalmology*, *107*(3), 450-456. https://doi.org/10.1016/S0161-6420(99)00024-X.

Das, D.K., Mukherjee, S., & Ray, D. (2011). Erratum to: resveratrol and red wine, healthy heart and longevity. *Heart failure reviews*, *16*(4), 425–435. https://doi.org/10.1007/s10741-011-9234-6.

D'Elia, L., Barba, G., Cappuccio, F.P., & Strazzullo, P. (2011). Potassium intake, stroke, and cardiovascular disease a meta-analysis of prospective studies. *Journal of the American College of Cardiology*, *57*(10), 1210–1219. https://doi.org/10.1016/j.jacc.2010.09.070.

Dherani, M., Murthy, G.V.S., Gupta, S.K., et al. (2008). Blood Levels of Vitamin C, Carotenoids and Retinol Are Inversely Associated with Cataract in a North Indian Population. *Investigative Ophthalmology & Visual Science*, *49*(8), 3328-3335. https://doi.org/10.1167/iovs.07-1202.

Engelgau, M.M., Geiss, L.S., Saadine, J.B., et al. (2004). The Evolving Diabetes Burden in the United States. *Annals of Internal Medicine*, *140*(11), 945-950. doi:10.7326/0003-4819-140-11-200406010-00035.

Fabiani, R., Minelli, L., & Rosignoli, P. (2016). Apple intake and cancer risk: a systematic review and meta-analysis of observational studies. *Public health nutrition*, *19*(14), 2603–2617. https://doi.org/10.1017/S136898001600032X.

Feeney, J., Finucane, C., et al. (2013). Low macular pigment optical density is associated with lower cognitive performance in a large, population-based sample of older adults. *Neurobiology of Aging, 34*(11), 2449-2456. https://doi.org/10.1016/j.neurobiolaging.2013.05.007.

Ferretti, G., Bacchetti, T., Belleggia, A., & Neri, D. (2010). Cherry antioxidants: from farm to table. *Molecules (Basel, Switzerland), 15*(10), 6993–7005. https://doi.org/10.3390/molecules15106993.

Feskanich, D., Ziegler, R.G., Michaud, D.S., et al. (2000). Prospective study of fruit and vegetable consumption and risk of lung cancer among men and women. *Journal of the National Cancer Institute, 92*(22), 1812–1823. https://doi.org/10.1093/jnci/92.22.1812.

Filaretova, L., & Bagaeva, T. (2016). The Realization of the Brain-Gut Interactions with Corticotropin-Releasing Factor and Glucocorticoids. *Current neuropharmacology, 14*(8), 876–881. https://doi.org/10.2174/1570159x14666160614094234.

Friedman, D.S., Wolfs, R.C., O'Colmain, B.J., Klein, B.E., et al (2004). Prevalence of open-angle glaucoma among adults in the United States. *Archives of ophthalmology (Chicago, Ill.: 1960), 122*(4), 532–538. https://doi.org/10.1001/archopht.122.4.532.

Fuerst, D.J., Tanzer, D.J., & Smith, R.E. (1998). Rheumatoid diseases. *International ophthalmology clinics, 38*(4), 47–80. https://doi.org/10.1097/00004397-199803840-00007.

Fujioka, K., Greenway, F., Sheard, J., & Ying, Y. (2006). The effects of grapefruit on weight and insulin resistance: relationship to the metabolic syndrome. *Journal of medicinal food, 9*(1), 49–54. https://doi.org/10.1089/jmf.2006.9.49.

Gagliardi, A., Totino, V., Cacciotti, F., Iebba, V., et al. (2018). Rebuilding the Gut Microbiota Ecosystem. *International journal of environmental research and public health, 15*(8), 1679. https://doi.org/10.3390/ijerph15081679.

Gajowik, A., & Dobrzyńska, M.M. (2014). Lycopene—antioxidant with radioprotective and anticancer properties. A review. *Roczniki Panstwowego Zakladu Higieny*, 65(4), 263–271. https://pubmed.ncbi.nlm.nih.gov/25526570/.

Green, K. (1998). Marijuana smoking vs cannabinoids for glaucoma therapy. *Archives of ophthalmology (Chicago, Ill.: 1960)*, 116(11), 1433–1437. https://doi.org/10.1001/archopht.116.11.1433.

Gutierrez, M.A., Davis, S.S., Rosko, A., Nguyen, S.M., et al. (2016). A novel AhR ligand, 2AI, protects the retina from environmental stress. *Scientific reports*, 6, 29025. https://doi.org/10.1038/srep29025.

Hecht S.S. (2000). Inhibition of carcinogenesis by isothiocyanates. *Drug metabolism reviews*, 32(3-4), 395–411. https://doi.org/10.1081/dmr-100102342.

Hill, D.A., & Artis, D. (2010). Intestinal bacteria and the regulation of immune cell homeostasis. *Annual review of immunology*, 28, 623–667. https://doi.org/10.1146/annurev-immunol-030409-101330.

Howatson, G., Bell, P.G., Tallent, J., Middleton, B., et al. (2012). Effect of tart cherry juice (Prunus cerasus) on melatonin levels and enhanced sleep quality. *European journal of nutrition*, 51(8), 909–916. https://doi.org/10.1007/s00394-011-0263-7.

Huxley, R., Lee, C.M., Barzi, F., et al. (2009). Coffee, decaffeinated coffee, and tea consumption in relation to incident type 2 diabetes mellitus: a systematic review with meta-analysis. *Archives of internal medicine*, 169(22), 2053–2063. https://doi.org/10.1001/archinternmed.2009.439.

Johnson, EJ. (2012). A possible role for lutein and zeaxanthin in cognitive function in the elderly. *The American Journal of Clinical Nutrition*, 96(5), 1161S-1165S.

Jonas, J.B., Wei, W.B., Xu, L., Rietschel, M., Streit, F., Wang Y.X. (2018). Self-rated depression and eye diseases: The Beijing Eye Study. *PLoS ONE*,

13(8): e0202132. https://doi.org/10.1371/journal.pone.0202132.

Jorde, R, Sneve, M, Figenschau, Y, et al. (2008). Effects of vitamin D supplementation on symptoms of depression in overweight and obese subjects: randomized double-blind trial. *Journal of Internal Medicine*, 264(6), 599-609. https://doi.org/10.1111/j.1365-2796.2008.02008.x.

Josling, P. (2001). Preventing the common cold with a garlic supplement: a double-blind, placebo-controlled survey. *Advances in therapy*, 18(4), 189–193. https://doi.org/10.1007/BF02850113.

Kang, F., Boland, M.V., Gupta, P., et al. (2016). Diabetes, Triglyceride Levels, and Other Risk Factors for Glaucoma in the National Health and Nutrition Examination Survey 2005–2008. Investigative Ophthalmology & Visual Science, 57(4), 2152-2157. https://doi.org/10.1167/iovs.15-18373.

Kang, J.H., Ascherio, A., Grodstein, F. (2005). Fruit and vegetable consumption and cognitive decline in aging women. *Annals of Neurology*, 57(5):713-720. https://doi.org/10.1002/ana.20476.

Kanny, D., Naimi, T.S., Liu, Y., et al. (2018). Annual Total Bing Drinks Consumed by U.S. Adults, 2015. *American Journal of Preventive Medicine*, 54(4), 486-396.

Kanthan, G.L., Mitchell, P., Burlutsky, G., et al. (2011). Fasting blood glucose levels and the long-term incidence and progression of cataract – the Blue Mountains Eye Study. *Acta Ophthalmologica*, 89(5), e434-e438. https://doi.org/10.1111/j.1755-3768.2011.02149.x.

Kaushik, S, Wang, JJ, Flood, V, et al. (2008). Dietary glycemic index and the risk of age-related macular degeneration, The American Journal of Clinical Nutrition, 88(4), 1104-1110. https://doi.org/10.1093/ajcn/88.4.1104.

Kelly, S.P., Thornton, J., Edwards, R., et al. (2005). Smoking and cataract: Review of causal association. *Journal of Cataract & Refractive Surgery*, 31(12), 2395-2404. https://doi.org/10.1016/j.jcrs.2005.06.039.

Kemeny-Beke, A., & Szodoray, P. (2020). Ocular manifestations of rheumatic diseases. *International ophthalmology, 40*(2), 503–510. https://doi.org/10.1007/s10792-019-01183-9.

Khurana, R.N., Porco, T.C., Claman, D.M., et al. (2016). Increasing Sleep Duration is Associated with Geographic Atrophy and Age-Related Macular Degeneration. *Retina: The Journal of Retinal and Vitreous Diseases, 36*(2), 255-258.

Klein, B.E., Knudtson, M.D., Lee, K.E., et al. (2008). Supplements and Age-Related Eye Conditions: The Beaver Dam Eye Study. *Ophthalmology, 115*(7), 1203-1208. https://doi.org/10.1016/j.ophtha.2007.09.011.

Knudtson, M.D., Klein, R., & Klein, B.E. (2006). Physical activity and the 15-year cumulative incidence of age-related macular degeneration: the Beaver Dam Eye Study. *The British journal of ophthalmology, 90*(12), 1461–1463. https://doi.org/10.1136/bjo.2006.103796.

Lam, C.T.Y., Trope, G.E., Buys, Y.M. (2017). Effect of Head Position and Weight Loss on Intraocular Pressure in Obese Subjects. *Journal of Glaucoma, 26*(2), 107-112.

Lenoir, M., Serre, F., Cantin, L., Ahmed, S.H. (2007). Intense Sweetness Surpasses Cocaine Reward. *PLoS ONE, 2*(8): e698. https://doi.org/10.1371/journal.pone.0000698.

Li, F., Hullar, M.A., Schwarz, Y., & Lampe, J.W. (2009). Human gut bacterial communities are altered by addition of cruciferous vegetables to a controlled fruit- and vegetable-free diet. *The Journal of nutrition, 139*(9), 1685–1691. https://doi.org/10.3945/jn.109.108191.

Li, Q., Han, Y., Dy, A., & Hagerman, R.J. (2017). The Gut Microbiota and Autism Spectrum Disorders. *Frontiers in cellular neuroscience, 11*, 120. https://doi.org/10.3389/fncel.2017.00120.
Littlejohns, TJ, Henley, WE, Lang, IA, et al. (2014). Vitamin D and the risk

of dementia and Alzheimer disease. *Neurology, 83*(10).

Lovallo, W.R., Wilson, M.F., Vincent, A.S., et al. (2004). Blood pressure response to caffeine shows incomplete tolerance after short-term regular consumption. *Hypertension (Dallas, Tex.: 1979), 43*(4), 760–765. https://doi.org/10.1161/01.HYP.0000120965.63962.93.

Lucas, M., Mirzaei, F., Pan, A., Okereke, O. I., et al. (2011). Coffee, caffeine, and risk of depression among women. *Archives of internal medicine, 171*(17), 1571–1578. https://doi.org/10.1001/archinternmed.2011.393.

Lukic, J., Chen, V., Strahinic, I., Begovic, J., et al. (2017). Probiotics or pro-healers: the role of beneficial bacteria in tissue repair. *Wound repair and regeneration: official publication of the Wound Healing Society [and] the European Tissue Repair Society, 25*(6), 912–922. https://doi.org/10.1111/wrr.12607.

Malik, V.S., Popkin, B.M., Bray, G.A., et al. (2010). Sugar-Sweetened Beverages and Risk of Metabolic Syndrome and Type 2 Diabetes. *Diabetes Care, 33*(11), 2477-2483. Retrieved from https://care.diabetesjournals.org/content/33/11/2477.short.

Mehrbod, P., Amini, E., Tavassoti-Kheiri, M. (2009). Antiviral activity of garlic extract on Influenza virus. *Iranian Journal of Virology, 1*(3), 19-23.

Meng, X., Li, Y., Li, S., Zhou, Y., Gan, R.Y., Xu, D.P., & Li, H.B. (2017). Dietary Sources and Bioactivities of Melatonin. *Nutrients, 9*(4), 367. https://doi.org/10.3390/nu9040367.

Menke, A., Casagrande, S., Geiss, L., Cowie, C.C. (2015). Prevalence of and Trends in Diabetes Among Adults in the United States, 1988-2012. JAMA, *314*(10), 1021–1029. doi:10.1001/jama.2015.10029.

Miserocchi, E., Fogliato, G., Modorati, G., & Bandello, F. (2013). Review on the worldwide epidemiology of uveitis. *European journal of ophthalmology, 23*(5), 705–717. https://doi.org/10.5301/ejo.5000278.

Molina-Levya, I., Molina-Levya, A., Bueno-Cavanillas, A. (2017). Efficacy of nutritional supplementation with omega-3 and omega-6 fatty acids in dry eye syndrome: a systematic review of randomized clinical trials. *Acta Ophthalmologica*, 95, e677–e685. Retrieved from https://onlinelibrary.wiley.com/doi/epdf/10.1111/aos.13428.

National Eye Institute. At a glance: Macular Edema. National Institutes of Health, July 28, 2019. Retrieved from https://www.nei.nih.gov/learn-about-eye-health/eye-conditions-and-diseases/macular-edema.

National Eye Institute. Diabetic Eye Disease Projected to Increase Among U.S. Population. National Institutes of Health, n.d. Retrieved from https://www.nei.nih.gov/sites/default/files/nehep-pdfs/GM_DED_drop-in%20article_2014.pdf.

Passo, M.S., Goldberg, L, Elliot, D.L., Van Buskirk, E.M. (1991). Exercise Training Reduces Intraocular Pressure Among Subjects Suspected of Having Glaucoma. Arch Ophthalmologica, *109*(8), 1096–1098. doi:10.1001/archopht.1991.01080080056027.

Pérez-Jiménez, J., Neveu, V., Vos, F., & Scalbert, A. (2010). Identification of the 100 richest dietary sources of polyphenols: an application of the Phenol-Explorer database. *European journal of clinical nutrition*, 64 Suppl 3, S112–S120. https://doi.org/10.1038/ejcn.2010.221.

Qui, M., Ramulu, P., Boland, M. (2019). Association Between Sleep Parameters and Glaucoma in the United States Population: National Health and Nutrition Examination Survey. *Journal of Glaucoma*, 28(2), 97-104.

Ramdas, W.D., Wolfs, R.C.W., Kiefte-de Jong, J.C., et al. (2012). Nutrient intake and risk of open-angle glaucoma: the Rotterdam Study. *European Journal of Epidemiology*, 27, 385–393. https://doi.org/10.1007/s10654-012-9672-z

Ravindran, R.D., Vashist, P., Gupta, S.K., et al. (2011). Inverse Association of Vitamin C with Cataract in Older People in India. *Ophthalmology, 118*(10), 1958-1965.e2. https://doi.org/10.1016/j.ophtha.2011.03.016.

Razak, M.A., Begum, P.S., Viswanath, B., & Rajagopal, S. (2017). Multifarious Beneficial Effect of Nonessential Amino Acid, Glycine: A Review. *Oxidative medicine and cellular longevity, 2017*, 1716701. https://doi.org/10.1155/2017/1716701.

Reddel, S., Putignani, L., & Del Chierico, F. (2019). The Impact of Low-FODMAPs, Gluten-Free, and Ketogenic Diets on Gut Microbiota Modulation in Pathological Conditions. *Nutrients, 11*(2), 373. https://doi.org/10.3390/nu11020373.

Renard, J.P., Rouland, J.F., Bron, A., et al. (2013). Nutritional, lifestyle and environmental factors in ocular hypertension and primary open-angle glaucoma: an exploratory case-control study. *Acta ophthalmologica, 91*(6), 505–513. https://doi.org/10.1111/j.1755-3768.2011.02356.x.

Ridley, N. J., Draper, B., & Withall, A. (2013). Alcohol-related dementia: an update of the evidence. *Alzheimer's research & therapy, 5*(1), 3. https://doi.org/10.1186/alzrt157.

Ried, K., Toben, C., & Fakler, P. (2013). Effect of garlic on serum lipids: an updated meta-analysis. *Nutrition reviews, 71*(5), 282–299. https://doi.org/10.1111/nure.12012.

Schleicher, M., Weikel, K., Garber, C., & Taylor, A. (2013). Diminishing risk for age-related macular degeneration with nutrition: a current view. *Nutrients, 5*(7), 2405–2456. https://doi.org/10.3390/nu5072405.

Schweiggert, R.M., Kopec, R.E., Villalobos-Gutierrez, M.G., Högel, J., et al. (2014). Carotenoids are more bioavailable from papaya than from tomato and carrot in humans: a randomised cross-over study. *The British journal of nutrition, 111*(3), 490–498. https://doi.org/10.1017/S0007114513002596.

Slavin, J. (2013). Fiber and prebiotics: mechanisms and health benefits. *Nu-

trients, 5(4), 1417–1435. https://doi.org/10.3390/nu5041417.

Snell, R.S., Lemp, M.A. (1998). *Clinical Anatomy of the Eye* (pp. 157-174). Malden: Blackwell Science, Inc.

Song, P., Wang, H., Theodoratou, E., Chan, K.Y., & Rudan, I. (2018). The national and subnational prevalence of cataract and cataract blindness in China: a systematic review and meta-analysis. *Journal of global health, 8*(1), 010804. https://doi.org/10.7189/jogh.08-010804.

Song, P., Xia, W., Wang, M., Chang, X., et al. (2018). Variations of Dry Eye Disease Prevalence by Age, Sex, and Geographic Characteristics in China: A Systematic Review and Meta-Analysis. *Journal of Global Health*, 2(8).

Stahre, M., Roeber, J., Kanny, D., Brewer, R. D., & Zhang, X. (2014). Contribution of excessive alcohol consumption to deaths and years of potential life lost in the United States. *Preventing chronic disease, 11*, E109. https://doi.org/10.5888/pcd11.130293.

St. Leger, A.S., Cochrane, A.L., Moore, F. (1979). Factors associated with cardiac mortality in developed countries with particular reference to the consumption of wine. *The Lancet, 8124*(313), 1017-1020. https://doi.org/10.1016/S0140-6736(79)92765-X.

Taylor, A., Jacques, P.F., Chylack, L.T., et al. (2002). Long-term intake of vitamins and carotenoids and odds of early age-related cortical and posterior subcapsular lens opacities. *The American Journal of Clinical Nutrition, 75*(3), 540-549. https://doi.org/10.1093/ajcn/75.3.540.

Taylor, A., Jacques, P.F., Nadler, D., et al. (1991). Relationship in humans between ascorbic acid consumption and levels of total and reduced ascorbic acid in lens, aqueous humor, and plasma. *Current Eye Research, 10*(8), 751-759. https://doi.org/10.3109/02713689109013869.

Thomson, M., Al-Qattan, K. K., Bordia, T., & Ali, M. (2006). Including garlic in the diet may help lower blood glucose, cholesterol, and triglycerides. *The*

Journal of nutrition, 136(3 Suppl), 800S–802S. https://doi.org/10.1093/jn/136.3.800S.

U.S. Department of Agriculture, Agricultural Research Service. FoodData Central, 2019.

U.S. Department of Health and Human Services and U.S. Department of Agriculture. 2015 – 2020 Dietary Guidelines for Americans. 8th Edition. December 2015. Available at https://health.gov/our-work/food-nutrition/previous-dietary-guidelines/2015.

Uzodike, E.B., Igwe, I.C. (2005). Efficacy of garlic (allium sativum) on staphylococcus aureus conjunctivitis. *Journal of Nigerian Optometric Association, 12*. Retrieved from https://www.ajol.info//index.php/jnoa/article/view/64453.

van Dieren, S., Uiterwaal, C.S.P.M., van der Schouw, Y.T., et al. (2009). Coffee and tea consumption and risk of type 2 diabetes. *Diabetologia* 52, 2561–2569. https://doi.org/10.1007/s00125-009-1516-3.

Wall H.K., Hannan J.A., Wright J.S. (2014). Patients With Undiagnosed Hypertension: Hiding in Plain Sight. JAMA, *312*(19), 1973–1974. doi:10.1001/jama.2014.15388.

Walsh, N.P., Fortes, M.B., Raymond-Barker, P., et al. (2012). Is Whole Body Hydration an Important Consideration in Dry Eye? *Investigative Ophthalmology and Visual Science, 53*(10), 6622-6627. https://doi.org/10.1167/iovs.12-10175.

Weickert, M.O., Pfeiffer, A.F.H. (2018). Impact of Dietary Fiber Consumption on Insulin Resistance and the Prevention of Type 2 Diabetes. *The Journal of Nutrition, 148*(1), 7-12.

Weikel, K.A., Garber, C., Baburins, A., & Taylor, A. (2014). Nutritional modulation of cataract. *Nutrition Reviews, 72*(1), 30–47. https://doi.org/10.1111/nure.12077.

West, S.K., Duncan, D.D., Muñoz, B., et al. (1998). Sunlight Exposure and Risk of Lens Opacities in a Population-Based Study: The Salisbury Eye Evaluation Project. JAMA, 280(8), 714–718. doi:10.1001/jama.280.8.714.

Wong, J., Lan, W., Ong, L.M., Tong, L. (2011). Non-hormonal Systemic Medications and Dry Eye. The Ocular Surface, 9(4), 212-226. https://doi.org/10.1016/S1542-0124(11)70034-9.

Yamadera, W., Inagawa, K., Chiba, S. et al. (2007). Glycine ingestion improves subjective sleep quality in human volunteers, correlating with polysomnographic changes. Sleep and Biological Rhythms, 5(2), 126-131. https://doi.org/10.1111/j.1479-8425.2007.00262.x.

Yang, Q., Zhang, Z., Gregg, E.W., Flanders, W.D., Merritt, R., Hu, F.B. (2014). Added Sugar Intake and Cardiovascular Diseases Mortality Among US Adults. JAMA Intern Med, 174(4), 516–524. doi:10.1001/jamainternmed.2013.13563.

Yeh, Y. Y., & Liu, L. (2001). Cholesterol-lowering effect of garlic extracts and organosulfur compounds: human and animal studies. The Journal of nutrition, 131(3s), 989S–93S. https://doi.org/10.1093/jn/131.3.989S.

Yuan, G.F., Sun, B., Yuan, J., & Wang, Q.M. (2009). Effects of different cooking methods on health-promoting compounds of broccoli. Journal of Zhejiang University. Science. B, 10(8), 580–588. https://doi.org/10.1631/jzus.B0920051.

Zhang, X., Shu, X.O., Xiang, Y.B., Yang, G., et al. (2011). Cruciferous vegetable consumption is associated with a reduced risk of total and cardiovascular disease mortality. The American journal of clinical nutrition, 94(1), 240–246. https://doi.org/10.3945/ajcn.110.009340.

Lightning Source UK Ltd.
Milton Keynes UK
UKHW050126250522
403405UK00004B/33/J